Clinical Experiences in Athletic Training

Kenneth L. Knight, PhD
Indiana State University

Human Kinetics Books

Library of Congress Cataloging-in-Publication Data

Knight, Kenneth L.
    Clinical experiences in athletic training / Kenneth L. Knight.
        p.   cm.
    Includes bibliographical references.
    ISBN 0-87322-289-X
    1. Physical education and training--Safety measures--Study and
teaching (Higher)   2. Sports--Accidents and injuries.   I. Title.
    GV344.K57   1990
    617.1'027--dc20   89-78029
                                                                       CIP

ISBN: 0-87322-289-X

Developmental Editor: Christine Drews; Copyeditor: Wendy Nelson; Assistant
Editors: Timothy Ryan, Valerie Hall, Robert King, and Julia Anderson; Proofreader:
Linda Siegel; Production Director: Ernie Noa; Typesetter: Angela K. Snyder;
Text Design: Keith Blomberg; Text Layout: Tara Welsch; Cover Design: Tim
Offenstein; Printer: United Graphics

Printed in the United States of America   10 9 8 7 6 5 4 3

Human Kinetics Books
A Division of Human Kinetics Publishers
P.O. Box 5076, Champaign, IL 61825-5076
1-800-747-4457

Canada: Human Kinetics Publishers, P.O. Box 24040, Windsor, ON N8Y 4Y9
1-800-465-7301 (in Canada only)

Europe: Human Kinetics Publishers (Europe) Ltd., P.O. Box IW14, Leeds LS16 6TR,
England
0532-781708

Australia: Human Kinetics Publishers, P.O. Box 80, Kingswood 5062, South Australia
618-374-0433

New Zealand: Human Kinetics Publishers, P.O. Box 105-231, Auckland 1
(09) 309-2259

Contents

Preface

Athletic training students must acquire practical skills. These skills require a knowledge base, but abstract knowledge is not enough—it must be applied. Skills necessary for competent sports injury management are developed only through clinical experience.

Usually the underlying assumption of clinical education in athletic training, and in many other medical fields, is that you learn by osmosis—that is, if you spend enough time ''on the job'' you will develop clinical skills by reacting to the situations you are exposed to there.

That approach is too haphazard. Students are not all exposed to the same injuries during their clinical experiences, and therefore they do not have equal opportunities to develop clinical skills. Another problem is that student athletic trainers often waste time during team practices. Typically there is a rush of activity immediately before practice as athletes are taped, bandaged, and cared for in preparation for the practice, and there is also much to do following practice. But unless an athlete is injured during the practice, many student athletic trainers spend practice time waiting for something to happen. If they are properly directed, student athletic trainers can use this time to develop and refine skills.

As a result, a plan was developed to ensure that all students can develop and demonstrate their competence in those clinical skills I feel are basic to the athletic training profession, whether or not they are exposed to the situations requiring those skills during their clinical experiences. The result of these efforts is the *Clinical Experiences in Athletic Training* modular program. The key is to ensure that each student athletic trainer is properly directed. The modular program does this.

Each module contains instructions for the student to develop specific skills, practice them on a peer, and then demonstrate his or her competence to a module supervisor.

Modules are arranged so that students begin developing simple skills and progressively acquire more complex ones. They are arranged into three levels and subgrouped within those levels, based

in part on the difficulty and complexity of the skills involved. Basic skills developed during many Level 1 modules are parts of more complex skills required for Level 2 modules.

The modules are also ordered according to a philosophy shared by many athletic training educators concerning the order in which knowledge and skills are developed. We have designed our curriculum so that, for all 4 years of their college experience, students take athletic training theory courses wherein they are taught the background information upon which skills are based. Students' clinical experience is limited to observation during their 2nd year and to actual working with the athletes during their 3rd and 4th years.

We have been using the module program since 1985 and have been pleased with students' skill development. Some athletic training educators and clinicians may desire a different progression; this can easily be achieved, and this book makes provisions for adapting the program to differing philosophies.

Most modules are totally generic, applying to students from any university. Others, which discuss filling out training room records and becoming familiar with local hospitals and physicians' offices, are specific to each university. Procedures have been incorporated that allow specific modules to be customized to each university's situation (see pp. 2-3). If necessary, individual institutions may add additional modules to meet their needs and specific philosophies.

Another advantage of the modular program is that it provides an additional guideline for assigning students to specific responsibilities. Athletic training instructors will have little worry when a Level 3 student has to perform without a staff athletic trainer present, because a Level 3 student has progressed through all levels of basic athletic training skills.

Conscious adherence to the program will result in students' mastering most of the skills identified for athletic trainers by the *NATA Role Delineation Study*. All skills under that study's Domains 1 through 4 (injury prevention, evaluation, management, and rehabilitation), as well as most under Domain 5 (organization and administration) and many under Domain 6 (education and counseling), will be developed by students progressing through this modularized clinical education program.

The modular program is effective for students in NATA-approved curriculum programs and in internship programs. Although students in internship programs spend more time in the training room, the extra clinical time does not ensure they will have greater exposure to injury situations. They need guidance and direction, as do curriculum students. The references at the back of the book will direct internship students to sources for obtaining the required background knowledge for each module.

This modularized approach to clinical education gives structure and objectivity to the process of developing clinical skills. Athletic training educators and students can be assured that those who have properly completed the program will have had at least laboratory experience in dealing with the most common athletic injuries. Thus it eliminates the ''hit or miss'' approach to most clinical education.

This project has been influenced by a number of colleagues; I gratefully acknowledge their contributions. Al Peppard used a competency-based approach with our students at the State University of New York College at Brockport. Katie Grove shared my frustration concerning clinical education of our students at Indiana State University and helped me outline the basis of this program. Vince Stilger and Bob Behnke of ISU, Jim Rankin of the University of Toledo, and Chris Ingersol of the University of Nevada–Las Vegas have used the program for the past 3 to 5 years; their comments and criticisms have helped. I also must acknowledge my introduction to modularized learning through the Weber State College WIL-kit program and the student who, years ago, came into my training room, sat in a corner twiddling his thumbs for 1-1/2 hours, got up, announced—more concerned with putting in time than mastering skills—that he had completed 600 hours (the requirement for certification at that time), and left.

The actual production of this book was enhanced by the enthusiasm for the project expressed by Bob Behnke of the NATA Professional Education Committee, Paul Grace of the NATA Board of Certification, and Rainer Martens of Human Kinetics Publishers. And my developmental editor, Chris Drews, has been a joy to work with.

Kenneth L. Knight

Using This Workbook

This book contains a structured but flexible program designed to guide you through experiences that will help you develop the skills and background necessary to be a competent athletic trainer. This program will direct and assist you in making practical application of the knowledge gained in theory classes. If you are not in an NATA curriculum program, you may have to spend extra time studying background material that curriculum students get in formal classes. References for background material are provided at the end of this manual.

The program contains modules that you will work on at your own pace. However, there are a minimum and a maximum number of modules that you should complete each semester. It is the intent of the program that most of the time you spend working on the modules (both developing the skills and demonstrating your competence) should be during regular training room hours; you should work with other students during "slack times." Your work on modules must not interfere with your training room duties, but you will have a great deal of time to work on them during team meetings, practices, and so on.

Each module consists of a list of competencies and explanations of what you must do to demonstrate mastery of those competencies. References are provided at the back of the book for most module competencies; these will help you refresh your knowledge of the material upon which the competency is based.

Module Progression

Modules are arranged into three levels and in blocks of related subject matter (designated by letters) within each level. X modules involve observation or working in an actual clinical setting; other modules involve developing specific clinical skills. The subject matter of each block of modules and the number of modules in that block follow.

Level 1 Modules

X1—Direct Clinical Experience (Observation) (2 modules)

A—Policies and Procedures (2 modules)

B—Emergency Procedures (3 modules)

C—Modality Operation (8 modules)

D—Advanced Modality Operation (9 modules)

E—Taping, Wrapping, Bracing, and Padding (8 modules)

F—Application to Program (1 module)

Level 2 Modules

X—Direct Clinical Experience (Team Rotation and Surgical Observation) (7 modules)

S—Supervision (1 module)

G—Management of Specific Injuries (15 modules)

H—Examination (Oral/Practical) (1 module)

Level 3 Modules

X—Direct Clinical Experience (Team Trainer and Internship) (2 modules)

S—Supervision (2 modules)

X modules involve direct clinical experiences. During Level 1 X modules you are assigned to the athletic training room (or rooms, if your college has more than one) to observe activities there. During Level 2 X modules you are assigned to work with a variety of teams as a student staff athletic trainer; these experiences will help you to learn the health care needs of various athletes and athletic teams. Your two Level 3 experiences will involve assignment to a single athletic team for the duration of their season; during these experiences you will apply and polish all the basic sports injury management skills you have learned and develop administrative and counseling skills.

During S modules you supervise and teach younger students. In so doing you review and solidify knowledge and skills you gained previously.

Modules within a block (i.e., with a similar prefix) can be worked on simultaneously and completed and approved in any order. All modules within each block must be completed before you can move on to the next block. Two exceptions are that *S* and *X* modules should be completed while working on other modules within the same level.

This modular rotation is based on a 3-year clinical rotation involving 1 year of observation and developing basic skills (Level 1) and 2 years of working directly with athletes and developing more complex skills (Levels 2 and 3). This is the preferred method for curriculum students, who take athletic training courses during each of their 4 years in college and progress through the modules during their sophomore through senior years.

An alternative progression based on a 4-year rotation is preferred for internship students, who usually begin providing athletic training services their first year in college, and those curriculums that have a 4-year rotation. The following is one possible outline of a 4-year progression.

Level 1 First-Year Modules

X1—Direct Clinical Experience (Observation) (1 module)

A—Policies and Procedures (2 modules)

B—Emergency Procedures (3 modules)

C—Modality Operation (8 modules)

E1—Taping, Wrapping, Bracing, and Padding (Ankle Taping and Wrapping) (1 module)

Level 1 Second-Year Modules

X2—Direct Clinical Experience (Observation) (1 module)

D—Advanced Modality Operation (9 modules)

E2 through E8—Taping, Wrapping, Bracing, and Padding (7 modules)

F—Application to Program (1 module)

Level 2 Modules

X3 through X8—Direct Clinical Experience (Team Rotation) (6 modules)

G—Management of Specific Injuries (15 modules)

X9—Direct Clinical Experience (Surgical Observation) (1 module)

S1—Supervision (1 module)

H—Examination (Oral/Practical) (1 module)

Level 3 Modules

X10 and X11—Direct Clinical Experience (Team Trainer and Internship) (2 modules)

S2 and S3—Supervision (2 modules)

Check with your athletic training program director or head athletic trainer to see whether he or she prefers a progression different from either of these.

Customizing Modules

Most modules are general and apply to all clinical settings. Others, however, are specific to each university setting. Those that are specific are listed here, along with the space needed to "customize" the module to your specific clinical setting.

Your athletic training curriculum director or head athletic trainer can supply you with the appropriate information for the modules listed. He or she may have photocopied this page from a previous student's book, written the information onto it, and then photocopied copies of the completed sheet. If so, time has been saved for both of you. If not, get the needed information from him or her.

INFORMATION FOR CUSTOMIZING MODULES

Module A2

All records and forms used in your training rooms, such as daily treatment logs, individual treatment sheets, insurance forms, referral to physician, and so on.

_____

_____

_____

_____

_____

_____

_____

_____

Module B3

Names of community medical services to which student athletic trainers may need to transport athletes, such as physicians' offices, hospital emergency rooms, hospital outpatient surgical units, and so on.

_____

_____

_____

_____

_____

_____

_____

Module C6

Weight training equipment that student athletic trainers will be using in your training rooms for rehabilitation. Include at least one piece for each of the major joints of the body.

ankle

_____

_____

knee

_____

_____

hip

_____

_____

shoulder

_____

_____

elbow

_____

_____

hand/wrist

_____

_____

Some modules in this book may not apply to your athletic training program, and there may be additional modules that your curriculum director or head athletic trainer has written specifically for you. These either are listed here or can be obtained from your curriculum director or head athletic trainer.

MODULES TO IGNORE

NAMES OF ADDITIONAL MODULES TO INCLUDE

Add these modules to the Level 1 and Level 2 master files found on pages 5 and 7, respectively.

C9 _____

C10 _____

D10 _____

D11 _____

E9 _____

E10 _____

G16 _____

G17 _____

Module Completion

You may demonstrate your mastery of module competencies during regular training room work hours. You should make arrangements ahead of time with an appropriate module supervisor. Allow extra time in case an emergency arises that would require your or your supervisor's services in caring for athletes. Before your conference with a module supervisor, check the references at the end of this book, practice the individual skills of the module, and then practice demonstrating all module skills to a peer. Also read the next section, "Tips for Module Supervisors," so that you will understand what is required of you.

Module supervisors include athletic training faculty and students at your college. Students may supervise and sign for module work at a level they have completed. A person at Level 3 can supervise people working on Levels 1 and 2; persons at Level 2 can supervise people at Level 1.

It is important that you begin getting modules checked off early in the semester. To prevent students from putting things off until the last minute, many programs have a policy that no more than two Level 1 modules or one Level 2 module may be completed per week during the last 5 weeks of the semester, and that no modules can be completed after Tuesday of the last week of the semester. Find out whether your program has such a policy.

After you successfully complete a module, the supervisor will sign and date the bottom of your workbook page and also sign and date your module master file (see pp. 5-8). On a regular basis, determined by your curriculum director or head athletic trainer, you will turn in the module master file sheet so that he or she can initial it. You will then have a double record of completed modules, one on the specific module sheet and one on the master file.

Tips for Module Supervisors

The success of the modular program, and the level of competence of younger students, depends on your competence as a module supervisor. In addition, as you demonstrate more competence as a supervisor your own knowledge and skill level will increase. Perhaps you have heard the phrase, "There is no better teacher than teaching someone else." The better a teacher you become, the greater your skills will become.

Your task is twofold: to help other students develop their skills and to verify module completion. Be liberal with your advice, but don't let students use you as their primary background source. Talk with them about what they have read concerning the topic. Make sure they have consulted at least two or three of the sources referenced at the end of this book, and encourage them to seek other sources. Use the sources yourself as you work with students—this will serve as an example to them as well as help you to be more accurate, which will increase your confidence.

Apply the following principles as students demonstrate their skill competencies to you:

- Check the comments section of the module before working with a student to make sure she or he is eligible.
- Remember to follow your program's policy concerning the number of modules students can complete during a calendar week, and also verify that all are completed within the required time limit.
- Make students actually demonstrate the skills. Some will have a tendency to tell you how they would do something. That is not enough. The phrase "I would . . ." has no place in completing modules. The student *must perform* the required tasks.
- Be fair with students—don't be too tough or too lenient. Letting a student slide through without really knowing the material is unfair to the student and to the program. All students will eventually be in a position of responsibility and must possess the necessary skills. On the other hand, being unreasonably difficult may discourage some students.
- All tasks of a specific module must be passed at the same time. A student who misses a single task must return another day and complete the entire module.
- A student who unsuccessfully attempts to pass a module cannot attempt that module again on the same day, either with the same or with a different module supervisor. Record, date, and initial unsuccessful attempts in the comments section at the end of the module.
- After a student successfully completes a module, sign and date *both* the individual module page and the module master file.

MASTER FILE—LEVEL 1

Name _____

Campus phone _____ Campus address_____

Permanent phone _____ Permanent address _____

Date clinical education started _____

Date accepted into/rejected from program _____

Semesters enrolled in clinical education _____

	Module	Date Completed	Evaluator	Comments
X1	Training Room Observation 1			
X2	Training Room Observation 2			
A1	Training Room Policies and Procedures			
A2	Training Room Records			
B1	ICES Application			
B2	CPR, Stretchers, and Splints			
B3	Medical Services (Health Centers, Hospitals, Physicians)			
C1	Cryokinetics Routine			
C2	Cryostretch Routine			
C3	Whirlpool Application			
C4	Hydrocollator Pack Application			
C5	DAPRE Routine for Knee, Ankle, and Shoulder			
C6	Isotonic Strength Training Devices			
C7	Therapeutic Use of a Stationary Bicycle			
C8	Pool Therapy			
C9	_____			
C10	_____			
D1	Ultrasound Application			
D2	Diathermy Application			
D3	Low Volt Electrical Muscle Stimulator Application			
D4	High Volt Electrical Muscle Stimulator Application			

(Cont.)

	Module	Date Completed	Evaluator	Comments
D5	TENS Application			
D6	Compression Devices	_____	_____	_____
D7	Isokinetic Devices	_____	_____	_____
D8	Manual Resistance Exercise Routines—Upper Extremity	_____	_____	_____
D9	Manual Resistance Exercise Routines—Lower Extremity	_____	_____	_____
D10	_____	_____	_____	_____
D11	_____	_____	_____	_____
E1	Ankle Taping and Wrapping	_____	_____	_____
E2	Knee Taping, Wrapping, and Bracing	_____	_____	_____
E3	Thigh and Lower Leg Taping, Wrapping, and Padding	_____	_____	_____
E4	Foot Care, Taping, Bracing, and Padding	_____	_____	_____
E5	Hip and Abdomen Taping and Wrapping	_____	_____	_____
E6	Shoulder Taping, Wrapping, and Bracing	_____	_____	_____
E7	Elbow-to-Wrist Taping, Wrapping, and Bracing	_____	_____	_____
E8	Hand and Finger Taping and Wrapping	_____	_____	_____
E9	_____	_____	_____	_____
E10	_____	_____	_____	_____
F1	Application to Athletic Training Program	_____	_____	_____

MASTER FILE—LEVEL 2

Name _____

Campus phone _____ Campus address_____

Permanent phone _____ Permanent address _____

Date clinical education started _____

Date accepted into/rejected from program _____

Semesters enrolled in clinical education _____

	Module	Date Completed	Evaluator	Comments
X3	Football Team Experience	_____	_____	_____
X4	Basketball Team Experience	_____	_____	_____
X5	Men's Team Sport Experience	_____	_____	_____
X6	Women's Team Sport Experience	_____	_____	_____
X7	Men's Individual Sport Experience	_____	_____	_____
X8	Women's Individual Sport Experience	_____	_____	_____
X9	Surgical Observation	_____	_____	_____
S1	Student Athletic Training Supervision	_____	_____	_____
G1	Foot Injury Management	_____	_____	_____
G2	Ankle Injury Management	_____	_____	_____
G3	Lower Leg Injury Management	_____	_____	_____
G4	Knee Injury Management	_____	_____	_____
G5	Thigh Injury Management	_____	_____	_____
G6	Hip and Groin Injury Management	_____	_____	_____
G7	Low Back Injury Management	_____	_____	_____
G8	Chest and Abdominal Injury Management	_____	_____	_____
G9	Shoulder Injury Management	_____	_____	_____
G10	Arm and Elbow Injury Management	_____	_____	_____
G11	Wrist and Hand Injury Management	_____	_____	_____
G12	Head and Neck Injury Management	_____	_____	_____
G13	Facial Injury Management	_____	_____	_____

(Cont.)

MASTER FILE—LEVEL 2 (Continued)

Module	Date Completed	Evaluator	Comments
G14 Management of Dermatological Conditions	_____	_____	_____
G15 Management of Common Illnesses	_____	_____	_____
G16 _____	_____	_____	_____
G17 _____	_____	_____	_____
H1 Oral/Practical Examination	_____	_____	_____

MASTER FILE—LEVEL 3

Name _____

Campus phone _____ Campus address_____

Permanent phone _____ Permanent address _____

Date clinical education started _____

Date accepted into/rejected from program _____

Semesters enrolled in clinical education _____

Module	Date Completed	Evaluator	Comments
X10 Team Trainer	_____	_____	_____
X11 Internship (Field Experience)	_____	_____	_____
S2 Student Athletic Training Supervision	_____	_____	_____
S3 Administration of Oral/Practical Examination	_____	_____	_____

Level 1

Training Room Observation 1

Competencies

1. Spend at least 70 hours observing the activities and operation of an athletic training room. You will be assigned specific times that you are to attend, and the assignment may be to different training rooms if your college has more than one.

2. Write two case reports during these experiences. Each report should cover 3 weeks and contain the pertinent events and information concerning an athlete's injury. In each report, include dates and specific details about the

   - injury,
   - immediate care,
   - rehabilitation, and
   - return to competition.

   Write both case studies in the form of a journal manuscript. See the "Guide to Contributors" section of *Athletic Training, Journal of the National Athletic Trainers Association*, for specific guidelines and tips.

3. Write an essay about the insights you have gained during this experience concerning athletic training as a profession. Turn in two copies of this essay; one will be returned to you, and the other will become part of your permanent athletic training file.

Grade _____ Date _____ Approved by _____

Comments:

Training Room Observation 2

Competencies

1. Spend at least 70 hours observing the activities and operation of an athletic training room. You will be assigned specific times that you are to attend, and the assignment may be to different training rooms if your college has more than one.
2. Write two case reports during these experiences. Each report should cover 3 weeks and contain the pertinent events and information concerning an athlete's injury. In each report, include dates and specific details about the

   • injury,
   • immediate care,

   • rehabilitation, and
   • return to competition.

   Write both case studies in the form of a journal manuscript. See the "Guide to Contributors" section of *Athletic Training, Journal of the National Athletic Trainers Association*, for specific guidelines and tips.
3. Write an essay about the insights you have gained during this experience concerning athletic training as a profession. Mention ideas and perceptions developed during Module X1 that have been strengthened and those that have been weakened. Turn in two copies of this essay; one will be returned to you, and the other will become part of your permanent athletic training file.

Grade _____ Date _____ Approved by _____
Comments:

Training Room Policies and Procedures

Competencies

1. Discuss the policies and procedures of each athletic training facility at your university. In your discussion, include the
   - location of the facility,
   - primary purpose or goal of the facility,
   - time (dates and time of day) of operation of the facility, and
   - faculty and student supervisors of the facility.
2. Describe the duties and responsibilities of each group of faculty/staff and student ath-

letic trainers involved in clinical experience at your university.
3. Discuss daily and weekly cleaning and maintenance responsibilities of student athletic trainers at each athletic training facility.

Mastery and Demonstration

Master these competencies through study, consultation with a Level 2 or 3 student, and practice on your own and with other Level 1 students. Then demonstrate your competence to a faculty member, a Level 2 student, or a Level 3 student.

Practice

	Date	Partner		Comments
1.	_____	_____		
2.	_____	_____		

Grade _____ Date _____ Approved by _____

Comments:

Training Room Records

Competencies

1. In the following spaces, write the specific names of the records listed on page 2. For each of these records, discuss the purpose of the record, demonstrate how to properly fill it out, and discuss where and for how long it is filed.

_____   _____

_____   _____

_____   _____

_____   _____

_____   _____

Mastery and Demonstration

Master these competencies through study, consultation with a Level 2 or 3 student, and practice on your own and with other Level 1 students. Then demonstrate your competence to a faculty member, a Level 2 student, or a Level 3 student.

Practice

	Date	Partner	Comments
1.	_____	_____	
2.	_____	_____	

Grade _____ Date _____ Approved by _____
Comments:

ICES Application

Competencies

1. Demonstrate application of *ice, compression, elevation, and support (ICES)* to an athlete with a sprained ankle, a dislocated finger, and a dislocated shoulder (three separate injuries). Indicate how long each would be applied, criteria for removal, reapplication, and so on.

2. Demonstrate your ability to assist an athlete to use crutches by properly fitting the crutches, instructing the athlete in proper crutch walking technique (both swing and three-point gaits), coach the athlete as he or she practices walking, and correct the athlete as necessary. Tell when to use each gait and how to help an athlete progress to normal walking.

3. Demonstrate application of two different types of slings (one with a triangular bandage, one with elastic wraps) to an athlete with a dislocated shoulder.

Mastery and Demonstration

Master these competencies through study, consultation with a Level 2 or 3 student, and practice on your own and with other Level 1 students. Then demonstrate your competence to a faculty member, a Level 2 student, or a Level 3 student.

Practice

	Date	Partner	Comments
1.	_____	_____	
2.	_____	_____	

Grade _____ Date _____ Approved by _____

Comments:

CPR, Stretchers, and Splints

Competencies

1. Demonstrate your competence in cardio-pulmonary resuscitation (CPR) either by having a valid American Red Cross or American Heart Association CPR card or by performing the technique on someone.
2. Explain the procedure for obtaining emergency care for

   • an athlete at your university and
   • a university student who is not an athlete.
3. Demonstrate proper use of a stretcher, a spine board and stretcher, and transportation off the field without a stretcher (e.g., for a sprained ankle or knee).

4. Demonstrate proper application of air splints for a dislocated talus and for the following fractures: middle of humerus, distal radius, distal fibula.

Mastery and Demonstration

Master these competencies through study, consultation with a Level 2 or 3 student, and practice on your own and with other Level 1 students. Then demonstrate your competence to a faculty member, a Level 2 student, or a Level 3 student.

Practice

	Date	Partner	Comments
1.	_____	_____	
2.	_____	_____	

Grade _____ Date _____ Approved by _____
Comments:

Medical Services
(Health Centers, Hospitals, Physicians)

Competencies

1. Complete a tour of your university student health center, hospital, or clinic where athletes are cared for. Have the person conducting the tour sign below. In addition, write the name of each of the following health center personnel. (Note: Check to see if any of these positions have different titles at your university. If so, replace the title of the position below with the proper one before the tour.)

Tour Director _____

Health Center Director _____

Assistant Director _____

Physician _____

Physician _____

Physician _____

Pharmacist _____

Head Nurse _____

Assistant Head Nurse _____

2. Visit the following community medical services and obtain the name and signature of the receptionist on duty (get the names of these medical services from page 3).

Facility	*Name/signature*
_____	_____
_____	_____
_____	_____
_____	_____
_____	_____
_____	_____
_____	_____
_____	_____
_____	_____

Module B3—Medical Services (Continued)

Facility

Name/signature

_____ _____

_____ _____

_____ _____

Grade _____ Date _____ Approved by _____

Comments:

Cryokinetics Routine

Competencies

1. Define *cryokinetics* and briefly explain
   - why it is used,
   - its effects,
   - its advantages,
   - its disadvantages,
   - its indications
   - its contraindications, and
   - precautions.
2. Demonstrate and explain cryokinetic
   - preapplication procedures,
   - application procedures, and
   - postapplication procedures.

3. Demonstrate proper recording of treatment on training room forms.

Mastery and Demonstration

Master these competencies through study, consultation with a Level 2 or 3 student, and practice on your own and with other Level 1 students. Then demonstrate your competence to a faculty member, a Level 2 student, or a Level 3 student.

Practice

	Date	Partner	Comments
1.	_____	_____	
2.	_____	_____	

Grade _____ Date _____ Approved by _____

Comments:

Cryostretch Routine

Competencies

1. Define *cryostretch* and briefly explain
   - why it is used,
   - its effects,
   - its advantages,
   - its disadvantages,
   - its indications,
   - its contraindications, and
   - precautions.
2. Demonstrate and explain cryostretch
   - preapplication procedures,
   - application procedures, and
   - postapplication procedures.

3. Demonstrate proper recording of treatment on training room forms.

Mastery and Demonstration

Master these skills through study, consultation with a Level 2 or 3 student, and practice on your own and with other Level 1 students. Then demonstrate your competence to a faculty member, a Level 2 student, or a Level 3 student.

Practice

	Date	Partner	Comments
1.	_____	_____	
2.	_____	_____	

Grade _____ Date _____ Approved by _____
Comments:

Whirlpool Application

Competencies

1. Define *whirlpool* and briefly explain
   - why it is used,
   - its effects,
   - its advantages,
   - its disadvantages,
   - its indications,
   - its contraindications, and
   - precautions.
2. Demonstrate and explain whirlpool
   - preapplication procedures,
   - application procedures, and
   - postapplication procedures.

3. Demonstrate and explain maintenance and simple repair procedures for whirlpools.
4. Demonstrate proper recording of treatment on training room forms.

Mastery and Demonstration

Master these skills through study, consultation with a Level 2 or 3 student, and practice on your own and with other Level 1 students. Then demonstrate your competence to a faculty member, a Level 2 student, or a Level 3 student.

Practice

	Date	Partner	Comments
1.	_____	_____	
2.	_____	_____	

Grade _____ Date _____ Approved by _____

Comments:

Hydrocollator Pack Application

Competencies

1. Describe a hydrocollator pack and briefly explain
   - why it is used,
   - its effects,
   - its advantages,
   - its disadvantages,
   - its indications,
   - its contraindications, and
   - precautions.
2. Demonstrate and explain hydrocollator pack
   - preapplication procedures,
   - application procedures, and
   - postapplication procedures.
3. Demonstrate and explain maintenance and simple repair procedures for hydrocollator packs.
4. Demonstrate proper recording of treatment on training room forms.

Mastery and Demonstration

Master these skills through study, consultation with a Level 2 or 3 student, and practice on your own and with other Level 1 students. Then demonstrate your competence to a faculty member, a Level 2 student, or a Level 3 student.

Practice

	Date	Partner	Comments
1.	_____	_____	
2.	_____	_____	

Grade _____ Date _____ Approved by _____

Comments:

DAPRE Routine for Knee, Ankle, and Shoulder

Competencies

1. Define *daily adjustable progressive resistive exercise (DAPRE)* and briefly explain the technique. Explain
   - why the technique was developed,
   - its advantages,
   - its disadvantages,
   - its indications,
   - its contraindications, and
   - precautions.
2. Explain the role of encouragement in use of the DAPRE technique. Demonstrate how you encourage an athlete.
3. Demonstrate and explain use of the DAPRE technique for
   - ankle rehabilitation,
   - knee rehabilitation, and
   - shoulder rehabilitation.
4. Demonstrate proper recording of treatment on training room forms.

Mastery and Demonstration

Master these skills through study, consultation with a Level 2 or 3 student, and practice on your own and with other Level 1 students. Then demonstrate your competence to a faculty member, a Level 2 student, or a Level 3 student.

Practice

	Date	Partner	Comments
1.	_____	_____	
2.	_____	_____	

Grade _____ Date _____ Approved by _____

Comments:

Isotonic Strength Training Devices

Competencies

1. Demonstrate proper use of the isotonic weight training equipment and conditions listed by doing each of the following:

   a. Set up the equipment.
   b. Position the patient.
   c. Stabilize the patient during repetitions.
   d. Demonstrate proper execution of repetitions (form, timing, control).
   e. Explain how and when to adjust the equipment.
   f. Demonstrate ways an athlete can "cheat" on the equipment.
   g. Outline safety factors for athlete and trainer.
   h. Demonstrate how to record results.

Equipment and Conditions

Ankle exerciser

Isotonic knee-thigh machine (for knee flexion and extension)

Isotonic machine weights for shoulder strengthening (abduction, internal and external rotation)

Free weight dumbbells for shoulder strengthening (abduction, internal and external rotation)

Mastery and Demonstration

Master these skills through study, consultation with a Level 2 or 3 student, and practice on your own and with other Level 1 students. Then demonstrate your competence to a faculty member, a Level 2 student, or a Level 3 student.

Practice

	Date	Partner		Comments
1.	_____	_____		
2.	_____	_____		

Grade _____ Date _____ Approved by _____
Comments:

Therapeutic Use of a Stationary Bicycle

Competencies

1. Explain and demonstrate each of the following (a-h) as they pertain to the use of a stationary bike for athletic injury care involving the conditions listed.

   a. Set up the equipment.
   b. Position the patient.
   c. Stabilize the patient during exercise.
   d. Properly execute the exercise (form, timing, control).
   e. Show how and when to make adjustments.
   f. Demonstrate ways an athlete can "cheat."
   g. Demonstrate safety factors for athlete and trainer.
   h. Demonstrate how to record treatments.

Conditions

Increasing joint range of motion
Developing muscular endurance
Developing cardiovascular endurance

Mastery and Demonstration

Master these skills through study, consultation with a Level 2 or 3 student, and practice on your own and with other Level 1 students. Then demonstrate your competence to a faculty member, a Level 2 student, or a Level 3 student.

Practice

	Date	Partner	Comments
1.	_____	_____	
2.	_____	_____	

Grade _____ Date _____ Approved by _____

Comments:

Pool Therapy

Competencies

1. Explain and demonstrate each of the following (a-h) as they pertain to the use of a swimming pool for athletic injury care involving the conditions listed.

   a. Explain special pool conditions such as depth of water, etc.
   b. Position the patient in the pool.
   c. Stabilize the patient during exercise.
   d. Properly execute the exercise (form, timing, control).
   e. Demonstrate how and when to make adjustments.
   f. Demonstrate ways an athlete can "cheat."
   g. Demonstrate safety factors for athlete and athletic trainer.
   h. Show how to record treatments.

Conditions

   Increasing joint range of motion
   Developing muscular endurance
   Developing cardiovascular endurance
   Relieving general muscular soreness
   Relieving general mental fatigue

Mastery and Demonstration

Master these skills through study, consultation with a Level 2 or 3 student, and practice on your own and with other Level 1 students. Then demonstrate your competence to a faculty member, a Level 2 student, or a Level 3 student.

Practice

	Date	Partner		Comments
1.	_____	_____		
2.	_____	_____		

Grade _____ Date _____ Approved by _____
Comments:

Ultrasound Application

Competencies

1. Define *ultrasound* and briefly explain
   - why it is used,
   - its therapeutic effects,
   - its advantages,
   - its disadvantages,
   - its indications,
   - its contraindications, and
   - precautions.

   In your discussion, include regular application, combined ultrasound and muscle stimulation, and phonophoresis.
2. Demonstrate and explain ultrasound
   - preapplication procedures,
   - application procedures, and
   - postapplication procedures.
3. Demonstrate and explain maintenance and simple repair procedures for ultrasounds.
4. Demonstrate proper recording of treatment on training room forms.

Mastery and Demonstration

Master these skills through study, consultation with a Level 2 or 3 student, and practice on your own and with other Level 1 students. Then demonstrate your competence to a faculty member, a Level 2 student, or a Level 3 student.

Practice

	Date	Partner	Comments
1.			
2.			

Grade _____ Date _____ Approved by _____

Comments:

Diathermy Application

Competencies

1. Describe diathermy and briefly explain
   - why it is used,
   - its effects,
   - its advantages,
   - its disadvantages,
   - its indications,
   - its contraindications, and
   - precautions.
2. Demonstrate and explain diathermy
   - preapplication procedures,
   - application procedures, and
   - postapplication procedures.

3. Demonstrate and explain maintenance and simple repair procedures for diathermy.
4. Demonstrate proper recording of treatment on training room forms.

Mastery and Demonstration

Master these skills through study, consultation with a Level 2 or 3 student, and practice on your own and with other Level 1 students. Then demonstrate your competence to a faculty member, a Level 2 student, or a Level 3 student.

Practice

	Date	Partner	Comments
1.	_____	_____	
2.	_____	_____	

Grade _____ Date _____ Approved by _____

Comments:

Low Volt Electrical Muscle Stimulator Application

Competencies

1. Define low volt muscle stimulation and briefly explain
   - why it is used,
   - its therapeutic effects,
   - its advantages,
   - its disadvantages,
   - its indications,
   - its contraindications, and
   - precautions.
2. Demonstrate and explain low volt muscle stimulation
   - preapplication procedures,
   - application procedures, and
   - postapplication procedures.

3. Demonstrate and explain maintenance and simple repair procedures for low volt muscle stimulation.
4. Demonstrate proper recording of treatment on training room forms.

Mastery and Demonstration

Master these skills through study, consultation with a Level 2 or 3 student, and practice on your own and with other Level 1 students. Then demonstrate your competence to a faculty member, a Level 2 student, or a Level 3 student.

Practice

	Date	Partner	Comments
1.	_____	_____	
2.	_____	_____	

Grade _____ Date _____ Approved by _____
Comments:

High Volt Electrical
Muscle Stimulator Application

Competencies

1. Define high volt twin pulse muscle stimulation and briefly explain

   - why it is used,
   - its effects,
   - its advantages,
   - its disadvantages,
   - its indications,
   - its contraindications, and
   - precautions.

2. Demonstrate and explain high volt muscle stimulation

   - preapplication procedures,
   - application procedures, and
   - postapplication procedures.

3. Demonstrate and explain maintenance and simple repair procedures for high volt muscle stimulators.
4. Demonstrate proper recording of treatment on training room forms.

Mastery and Demonstration

Master these skills through study, consultation with a Level 2 or 3 student, and practice on your own and with other Level 1 students. Then demonstrate your competence to a faculty member, a Level 2 student, or a Level 3 student.

Practice

	Date	Partner	Comments
1.	_____	_____	
2.	_____	_____	

Grade _____ Date _____ Approved by _____
Comments:

TENS Application

Competencies

1. Describe *transcutaneous electrical nerve stimulation* (TENS) and briefly explain

   - why it is used,
   - its effects,
   - its advantages,
   - its disadvantages,
   - its indications,
   - its contraindications, and
   - precautions.

2. Demonstrate and explain TENS

   - preapplication procedures,
   - application procedures, and
   - postapplication procedures.

3. Demonstrate and explain maintenance and simple repair procedures for a TENS unit.

4. Demonstrate proper recording of treatment on training room forms.

Mastery and Demonstration

Master these skills through study, consultation with a Level 2 or 3 student, and practice on your own and with other Level 1 students. Then demonstrate your competence to a faculty member, a Level 2 student, or a Level 3 student.

Practice

	Date	Partner		Comments
1.	_____	_____		
2.	_____	_____		

Grade _____ Date _____ Approved by _____

Comments:

Compression Devices

Competencies

1. Describe compression devices (such as Jobst) and briefly explain
   - why they are used,
   - their effects,
   - their advantages,
   - their disadvantages,
   - their indications,
   - their contraindications, and
   - precautions.
2. Demonstrate and explain compression device
   - preapplication procedures,
   - application procedures, and
   - postapplication procedures.
3. Demonstrate and explain maintenance and simple repair procedures for compression devices.
4. Demonstrate proper recording of treatment on training room forms.

Mastery and Demonstration

Master these skills through study, consultation with a Level 2 or 3 student, and practice on your own and with other Level 1 students. Then demonstrate your competence to a faculty member, a Level 2 student, or a Level 3 student.

Practice

	Date	Partner	Comments
1.	_____	_____	
2.	_____	_____	

Grade _____ Date _____ Approved by _____

Comments:

Isokinetic Devices

Competencies

1. Explain what isokinetic resistance is and how it is developed by the Orthotron, Cybex, KinCom, and Hydra Gym.
2. Explain differences among isokinetic programs for development of

   - strength,
   - speed,
   - power, and
   - endurance.

3. Demonstrate proper use of an isokinetic device for each of the conditions listed by doing each of the following:

   a. Set up equipment.
   b. Position the patient.
   c. Stabilize the patient during repetitions.
   d. Demonstrate proper execution of repetitions (form, timing, control).
   e. Explain how and when to adjust the equipment.
   f. Demonstrate ways an athlete can "cheat" on the equipment.
   g. Outline safety factors for athlete and trainer.
   h. Demonstrate how to record results.

Conditions

Knee rehabilitation
Shoulder rehabilitation

Mastery and Demonstration

Master these skills through study, consultation with a Level 2 or 3 student, and practice on your own and with other Level 1 students. Then demonstrate your competence to a faculty member, a Level 2 student, or a Level 3 student.

Practice

	Date	Partner	Comments
1.			
2.			

Grade _____ Date _____ Approved by _____

Comments:

Manual Resistance Exercise Routines—
Upper Extremity

Competencies

Demonstrate proper use of manual resistance and passive stretching exercises (PNF, Shelton exercise routines, etc.) for developing strength and range of motion by completing Competencies 1 through 3 for each of the following:

Neck

Shoulder girdle

Shoulder joint

Elbow

Forearm

Wrist

Fingers

1. Describe the objective of the manual resistance exercise routines for each body part listed, and briefly explain the advantages, disadvantages, indications, contraindications, and precautions for using the routine.
2. For each body part listed, demonstrate and explain the manual resistance exercise routine
   - preapplication procedures,
   - application procedures, and
   - postapplication procedures.
3. Demonstrate proper recording of manual resistance exercises on training room forms.

Mastery and Demonstration

Master these skills through study, consultation with a Level 2 or 3 student, and practice on your own and with other Level 1 students. Then demonstrate your competence to a faculty member, a Level 2 student, or a Level 3 student.

Practice

     Date   Partner   Comments

1. _____ _____

2. _____ _____

Grade _____ Date _____ Approved by _____

Comments:

Manual Resistance Exercise Routines— Lower Extremity

Competencies

Demonstrate proper use of manual resistance and passive stretching exercises (PNF, Shelton exercise routines, etc.) for developing strength and range of motion by completing Competencies 1 through 3 for each of the following:

Foot

Ankle

Knee

Quadriceps

Hamstring

Hip and groin

Abdomen

Low back

1. Describe the objective of the manual resistance exercise routines for each body part listed, and briefly explain the advantages, disadvantages, indications, contraindications, and precautions for using the routine.
2. For each body part listed, demonstrate and explain the manual resistance exercise routine
   - preapplication procedures,
   - application procedures, and
   - postapplication procedures.
3. Demonstrate proper recording of manual resistance exercises on training room forms.

Mastery and Demonstration

Master these skills through study, consultation with a Level 2 or 3 student, and practice on your own and with other Level 1 students. Then demonstrate your competence to a faculty member, a Level 2 student, or a Level 3 student.

Practice

	Date	Partner	Comments
1.	_____	_____	
2.	_____	_____	

Grade _____ Date _____ Approved by _____

Comments:

Ankle Taping and Wrapping

Competencies

The following tasks must be done correctly, quickly, and neatly.

1. Demonstrate your ability to apply the following wraps (cloth and elastic):

   - Ankle wrap (Illinois) and trace in less than 25 seconds
   - Ankle wrap (Louisiana) and trace in less than 25 seconds
   - Elastic wrap for post ankle sprain compression and support

2. Demonstrate your ability to apply the following ankle adhesive taping procedures:

   - A basic preventative in less than 2 minutes 45 seconds
   - A second type of basic preventative in less than 2 minutes 45 seconds
   - An extra support (for 2° injury) in less than 3 minutes 30 seconds

Mastery and Demonstration

Master these skills through study, consultation with a Level 2 or 3 student, and practice on your own and with other Level 1 students. Then demonstrate your competence to a faculty member, a Level 2 student, or a Level 3 student.

Practice

	Date	Partner	Comments
1.	_____	_____	
2.	_____	_____	

Grade _____ Date _____ Approved by _____
Comments:

Knee Taping, Wrapping, and Bracing

Competencies

The following tasks must be done correctly, quickly, and neatly.

1. Demonstrate your ability to apply elastic wraps for the following two conditions:
   - Post collateral knee injury support
   - Post hyperextension knee injury support
2. Demonstrate your ability to apply an accepted adhesive taping procedure to the following injuries:
   - Medial collateral knee ligament (medial and/or lateral)
   - Hyperextended knee
   - Improper patellar tracking

3. Demonstrate your ability to apply the following types of knee braces:
   - Lateral brace without neoprene
   - Lateral brace with neoprene
   - Post injury/surgery immobilization brace
   - Patellar tracking brace
   - Lenox Hill or other derotation brace

Mastery and Demonstration

Master these skills through study, consultation with a Level 2 or 3 student, and practice on your own and with other Level 1 students. Then demonstrate your competence to a faculty member, a Level 2 student, or a Level 3 student.

Practice

	Date	Partner	Comments
1.	_____	_____	
2.	_____	_____	

Grade _____ Date _____ Approved by _____
Comments:

Thigh and Lower Leg Taping, Wrapping, and Padding

Competencies

The following tasks must be done correctly, quickly, and neatly.

1. Demonstrate your ability to apply elastic wraps to a thigh strain.
2. Demonstrate your ability to apply an accepted adhesive taping procedure to the following injuries:
   - Achilles tendon sprain
   - Shin splints

3. Demonstrate your ability to apply pads for the following injuries:
   - Quadriceps contusion
   - Shin contusion

Mastery and Demonstration

Master these skills through study, consultation with a Level 2 or 3 student, and practice on your own and with other Level 1 students. Then demonstrate your competence to a faculty member, a Level 2 student, or a Level 3 student.

Practice

	Date	Partner	Comments
1.	_____	_____	
2.	_____	_____	

Grade _____ Date _____ Approved by _____
Comments:

Foot Care, Taping, Bracing, and Padding

Competencies

1. Demonstrate your ability to care for the following foot injuries:
   - Blister
   - Corns and bunions
   - Ingrown toenail

The following tasks must be done correctly, quickly, and neatly.

2. Demonstrate your ability to apply an accepted adhesive taping procedure to the following injuries:
   - Sprained hallicus
   - Sprained digit
   - Longitudinal arch
   - Contused calcaneal fat pad
   - Heel bruise

3. Demonstrate your ability to apply appropriate pads and braces for the following injuries:
   - Metatarsal stress fracture
   - Phalange fracture
   - Heel spur
   - Heel bruise

Mastery and Demonstration

Master these skills through study, consultation with a Level 2 or 3 student, and practice on your own and with other Level 1 students. Then demonstrate your competence to a faculty member, a Level 2 student, or a Level 3 student.

Practice

	Date	Partner	Comments
1.	_____	_____	
2.	_____	_____	

Grade _____ Date _____ Approved by _____

Comments:

Hip and Abdomen Taping and Wrapping

Competencies

The following tasks must be done correctly, quickly, and neatly.

1. Demonstrate your ability to apply elastic wraps to the following injuries:
   - Groin strain—adductors
   - Groin strain—flexors
2. Demonstrate your ability to apply an accepted adhesive taping procedure to the following injuries:
   - Sacroiliac sprain
   - Lumbosacral sprain
   - Hip pointer

3. Demonstrate your ability to apply a brace to a lumbosacral sprain.

Mastery and Demonstration

Master these skills through study, consultation with a Level 2 or 3 student, and practice on your own and with other Level 1 students. Then demonstrate your competence to a faculty member, a Level 2 student, or a Level 3 student.

Practice

	Date	Partner	Comments
1.	_____	_____	
2.	_____	_____	

Grade _____ Date _____ Approved by _____

Comments:

Shoulder Taping, Wrapping, and Bracing

Competencies

The following tasks must be done correctly, quickly, and neatly.

1. Demonstrate your ability to apply the following wraps:
   - Shoulder sling (cloth)
   - Shoulder sling (elastic wraps)
   - Shoulder spica
2. Demonstrate your ability to apply an accepted adhesive taping procedure to the following injuries:
   - Acromioclavicular sprain
   - Sternoclavicular sprain

3. Demonstrate your ability to apply the following braces:
   - Shoulder harness
   - Shoulder pads
   - AC brace

Mastery and Demonstration

Master these skills through study, consultation with a Level 2 or 3 student, and practice on your own and with other Level 1 students. Then demonstrate your competence to a faculty member, a Level 2 student, or a Level 3 student.

Practice

	Date	Partner	Comments
1.	_____	_____	
2.	_____	_____	

Grade _____ Date _____ Approved by _____

Comments:

Elbow-to-Wrist Taping, Wrapping, and Bracing

Competencies

The following tasks must be done correctly, quickly, and neatly.

1. Demonstrate your ability to apply elastic wraps to the following body parts or injuries:
   - Elbow contusion
   - Wrist (football)
   - Wrist (gymnast)
   - Wrist (double friction blister pad)

2. Demonstrate your ability to apply an accepted adhesive taping procedure to the following injuries:
   - Elbow hyperextension
   - Forearm splints

- Wrist flexor strain
- Wrist extensor strain

3. Demonstrate your ability to apply the braces for the following injuries:
   - Epicondylitis
   - Elecronan bursa contusion using sorbothane

Mastery and Demonstration

Master these skills through study, consultation with a Level 2 or 3 student, and practice on your own and with other Level 1 students. Then demonstrate your competence to a faculty member, a Level 2 student, or a Level 3 student.

Practice

	Date	Partner	Comments
1.	_____	_____	
2.	_____	_____	

Grade _____ Date _____ Approved by _____

Comments:

Hand and Finger Taping and Wrapping

Competencies

The following tasks must be done correctly, quickly, and neatly.

1. Demonstrate your ability to apply the following elastic and cloth wraps to the body parts listed:
   - Thumb with cloth wrap
   - Sprained finger with elastic tape
2. Demonstrate your ability to apply an accepted adhesive taping procedure to the following injuries:
   - Hand contusion
   - Hand sprain
   - Thumb sprain
   - Thumb sprain with reverse spica
   - PIP sprain
   - DIP sprain
   - Boutonniere
   - Finger dislocation
   - Finger hyperextension
   - Mallet finger

Mastery and Demonstration

Master these skills through study, consultation with a Level 2 or 3 student, and practice on your own and with other Level 1 students. Then demonstrate your competence to a faculty member, a Level 2 student, or a Level 3 student.

Practice

	Date	Partner	Comments
1.	_____	_____	
2.	_____	_____	

Grade _____ Date _____ Approved by _____
Comments:

Application to Athletic Training Program

Competencies

1. Make formal application to your athletic training program. Contact your athletic training curriculum director or head athletic trainer for application materials, deadlines, and so on.

Date application was obtained _____

Date application was completed _____

Level 2

Football Team Experience

Competencies

1. Work a minimum of 4 weeks and 100 hours with the football team as a student member of the athletic training staff.
2. Outline on paper and discuss with your supervisor the following:

   - The organization of athletic training services for the football team. Include the organization (i.e., type of equipment and staff members' functions) of the training room and field for practices and games.
   - Proper fitting of all required (by NCAA and High School AA) and optional equipment for football. Demonstrate this as well.
   - The skills and activities specific to football that lead to injury.
   - The most common football injuries.
   - Ways to prevent the most common football injuries.
   - NCAA and High School AA rules concerning taping and bandaging for games.
   - NCAA and High School AA rules concerning injury care during games.
   - The elements of successful pre-, in-, and postseason conditioning programs for football. Include activities that develop flexibility, strength, muscular endurance, speed, coordination, agility, power, and cardiorespiratory endurance.
   - The three to five athletes on the team who you feel perform their conditioning exercises most correctly, the three to five who perform them least correctly, and why you chose each.

Grade _____ Date _____ Approved by _____

Comments:

Basketball Team Experience

Competencies

1. Work a minimum of 4 weeks and 75 hours with either the men's or the women's basketball team as a student member of the athletic training staff.
2. Outline on paper and discuss with your supervisor the following:
   - The organization of athletic training services for the basketball team. Include the organization (i.e., type of equipment and staff members' functions) of the training room and court for practices and games.
   - Proper fitting of all required (by NCAA and High School AA) and optional equipment for basketball. Demonstrate this as well.
   - The skills and activities specific to basketball that lead to injury.
   - The most common basketball injuries.
   - Ways to prevent the most common basketball injuries.
   - NCAA and High School AA rules concerning taping and bandaging for basketball games.
   - NCAA and High School AA rules concerning injury care during basketball games.
   - Differences (from the athletic training point of view) between this sport and other sports you have worked.
   - The elements of successful pre-, in-, and postseason conditioning programs for basketball. Include activities that develop flexibility, strength, muscular endurance, speed, coordination, agility, power, and cardiorespiratory endurance.
   - The three athletes on the team who you feel perform their conditioning exercises most correctly, the three who perform them least correctly, and why you chose each.

Grade _____ Date _____ Approved by _____

Comments:

Men's Team Sport Experience

Competencies

1. Work a minimum of 4 weeks and 75 hours with a men's team sport (other than football or basketball) as a student member of the athletic training staff.
2. Outline on paper and discuss with your supervisor the following:

   - The organization of athletic training services for the team. Include the organization (i.e., type of equipment and staff members' functions) of the training room and the court or field for practices and games.
   - Proper fitting of all required (by NCAA and High School AA) and optional equipment for the team. Demonstrate this as well.
   - The skills and activities specific to this sport that lead to injury.
   - The most common injuries in this sport.
   - Ways to prevent the most common injuries in this sport.
   - NCAA and High School AA rules concerning taping and bandaging for this sport's contests.
   - NCAA and High School AA rules concerning injury care during this sport's contests.
   - Differences (from the athletic training point of view) between this sport and other sports you have worked.
   - The elements of successful pre-, in-, and postseason conditioning programs for this sport. Include activities that develop flexibility, strength, muscular endurance, speed, coordination, agility, power, and cardiorespiratory endurance.
   - The three to five athletes on the team who you feel perform their conditioning exercises most correctly and the three to five who perform them least correctly; explain why you chose each.

Grade _____ Date _____ Approved by _____

Comments:

Women's Team Sport Experience

Competencies

1. Work a minimum of 4 weeks and 75 hours with a women's team sport (other than basketball) as a student member of the athletic training staff.
2. Outline on paper and discuss with your supervisor the following:

   * The organization of athletic training services for the team. Include the organization (i.e., type of equipment and staff members' functions) of the training room and the court or field for practices and games.
   * Proper fitting of all required (by NCAA and High School AA) and optional equipment for the team. Demonstrate this as well.
   * The skills and activities specific to this sport that lead to injury.
   * The most common injuries in this sport.
   * Ways to prevent the most common injuries in this sport.
   * NCAA and High School AA rules concerning taping and bandaging for this sport's contests.
   * NCAA and High School AA rules concerning injury care during this sport's contests.
   * Differences (from the athletic training point of view) between this sport and other sports you have worked.
   * The elements of successful pre-, in-, and postseason conditioning programs for this sport. Include activities that develop flexibility, strength, muscular endurance, speed, coordination, agility, power, and cardiorespiratory endurance.
   * The three to five athletes on the team who you feel perform their conditioning exercises most correctly and the three to five who perform them least correctly; explain why you chose each.

Grade _____ Date _____ Approved by _____

Comments:

Men's Individual Sport Experience

Competencies

1. Work a minimum of 4 weeks and 75 hours as a student member of the athletic training staff for a men's team that involves individual sport competition (e.g., gymnastics or track and field).
2. Outline on paper and discuss with your supervisor the following:
   - The organization of athletic training services for the team. Include the organization (i.e., type of equipment and staff members' functions) of the training room and the court or field for practices and games.
   - Proper fitting of all required (by NCAA and High School AA) and optional equipment for the team. Demonstrate this as well.
   - The skills and activities specific to this sport that lead to injury.
   - The most common injuries in this sport.
   - Ways to prevent the most common injuries in this sport.
   - NCAA and High School AA rules concerning taping and bandaging for this sport's contests.
   - NCAA and High School AA rules concerning injury care during this sport's contests.
   - Differences (from the athletic training point of view) between this sport and other sports you have worked.
   - The elements of successful pre-, in-, and postseason conditioning programs for this sport. Include activities that develop flexibility, strength, muscular endurance, speed, coordination, agility, power, and cardiorespiratory endurance.
   - The three to five athletes on the team who you feel perform their conditioning exercises most correctly and the three to five who perform them least correctly; explain why you chose each.

Grade _____ Date _____ Approved by _____

Comments:

Women's Individual Sport Experience

Competencies

1. Work a minimum of 4 weeks and 75 hours as a student member of the athletic training staff for a women's team that involves individual sport competition (e.g., gymnastics or track and field).
2. Outline on paper and discuss with your supervisor the following:
   - The organization of athletic training services for the team. Include the organization (i.e., type of equipment and staff members' functions) of the training room and the court or field for practices and games.
   - Proper fitting of all required (by NCAA and High School AA) and optional equipment for the team. Demonstrate this as well.
   - The skills and activities specific to this sport that lead to injury.
   - The most common injuries in this sport.
   - Ways to prevent the most common injuries in this sport.
   - NCAA and High School AA rules concerning taping and bandaging for this sport's contests.
   - NCAA and High School AA rules concerning injury care during this sport's contests.
   - Differences (from the athletic training point of view) between this sport and other sports you have worked.
   - The elements of successful pre-, in-, and postseason conditioning programs for this sport. Include activities that develop flexibility, strength, muscular endurance, speed, coordination, agility, power, and cardiorespiratory endurance.
   - The three to five athletes on the team who you feel perform their conditioning exercises most correctly and the three to five who perform them least correctly; explain why you chose each.

Grade _____ Date _____ Approved by _____

Comments:

Surgical Observation

Competencies

1. Observe two different surgical procedures. With each, discuss with one of the physicians or a surgical nurse or technician the presurgical preparation of the patient and the procedures that will be followed for the first 12 to 24 hours after surgery.

2. Within 48 hours (the sooner the better) of the surgery, discuss the surgery with a module supervisor. Include in this discussion the rehabilitation procedures that this patient probably will follow.

Grade 1 _____ Date _____ Approved by _____

Grade 2 _____ Date _____ Approved by _____

Comments:

Student Athletic Training Supervision

Competencies

1. Work with at least five different Level 1 students on a total of 30 Level 1 modules. This includes reviewing material with them and testing them for their mastery of the material.

	Date	Person examined	Module	Grade given
1.				
2.				
3.				
4.				
5.				
6.				
7.				
8.				
9.				
10.				
11.				
12.				
13.				
14.				
15.				
16.				
17.				
18.				
19.				
20.				
21.				
22.				
23.				
24.				
25.				

26. _____ _____ _____ _____

27. _____ _____ _____ _____

28. _____ _____ _____ _____

29. _____ _____ _____ _____

30. _____ _____ _____ _____

Grade _____ Date _____ Approved by _____

Comments:

Foot Injury Management

Competencies

1. Name and palpate each of the following bones and any prominent features listed:
   - Calcaneous
   - Talus
   - Cuboid
   - Navicular
   - Cuneiforms
   - Metatarsals
     Styloid process of fifth
     Heads
   - Phalanges
   - Sesamoids

2. On someone other than yourself, palpate or draw the joint line, then perform active and passive joint range of motion tests, and tests to determine joint stability for each of the following articulations:
   - Subtalar
   - Transverse tarsal
   - Metatarsal-phangeal (MP)
   - Interphangeal (PIP and DIP)

3. Using surface anatomy, palpate or draw, on someone other than yourself, the origins and course of each of the following ligaments:
   - Long plantar
   - Lateral retanaculum

4. Using surface anatomy, palpate or draw, on someone other than yourself, the origin, insertion, and course of each of the following muscles. Then tell the major function of the muscle.
   - Anterior tibialis
   - Flexor hallicus longus
   - Flexor digitorum longus
   - Posterior tibialis
   - Extensor hallicus longus
   - Extensor digitorum longus
   - Peroneus longus
   - Peroneus brevis
   - Peroneus tertius
   - Gastrocnemius
   - Soleus

5. Demonstrate, on someone other than yourself, functional tests to determine the normalcy of each of the muscles and ligaments in Competencies 3 and 4. Use tests to determine the stability of the ligaments listed in Competency 3 and the flexibility and strength of the muscles listed in Competency 4.

6. Using surface anatomy, palpate, on someone other than yourself, each of the following structures:
   - Peroneal nerve (entire course)
   - Tibial nerve (entire course)
   - Pedal pulse

Use the following list of injuries to complete Competencies 7 through 11.

Ingrown toenail

Bunion

Calluses and corns

Blisters

Neuroma

Hammer toe

Sprained hallux

Sprained digit

Arch strains

Plantar fascitis

Heel bruise

Bursitis

Tenosynovitis

Fractures

Stress fractures

Avulsion fractures

Sinus tarsi syndrome

7. Explain and demonstrate the mechanisms by which each of the listed injuries occur. Name the three sports in which each injury is most likely to occur, and explain any differences among the injury occurrences/mechanisms in those sports.

8. Explain and demonstrate, on someone other than yourself, the appropriate immediate care procedures for each listed injury. Explain the objectives, and criteria for progressing, for each step in the procedure.

9. Demonstrate, on someone other than yourself, a complete rehabilitation program for each listed injury. As you proceed, explain the objectives and procedures of each step in the program. Explain the measurement criteria for advancing from one step to another.

10. Using pictures or illustrations, explain the objectives and procedures of prophylactic taping, padding, and bandaging for the listed injuries as appropriate.

11. Demonstrate or explain procedures for preventing each listed injury.

Mastery and Demonstration

Master these skills through study, consultation with a Level 3 student, and practice on your own and with other Level 2 students. Then demonstrate your competence to a faculty member or a Level 3 student.

Practice

     Date   Partner   Comments

1. _____ _____

2. _____ _____

Grade _____ Date _____ Approved by _____

Comments:

Ankle Injury Management

Competencies

1. Name and palpate each of the following bones and any prominent features listed:

   - Calcaneous
   - Talus
   - Cuboid
   - Navicular
   - Cuneiforms
   - Tibia
   - Fibula

2. On someone other than yourself, palpate or draw the joint line, then perform active and passive joint range of motion tests, and tests to determine joint stability for each of the following articulations:

   - Ankle mortice
   - Distal tibiofibular
   - Subtalar
   - Transverse tarsal

3. Using surface anatomy, palpate or draw, on someone other than yourself, the origins and course of each of the following ligaments:

   - Anterior talofibular
   - Calcaneofibular
   - Posterior talofibular
   - Distal anterior tibiofibular
   - Distal posterior tibiofibular
   - Deltoid
   - Lateral retanaculum

4. Using surface anatomy, palpate or draw, on someone other than yourself, the origin, insertion, and course of each of the following muscles. Then tell the major function of the muscle.

   - Anterior tibialis
   - Flexor hallicus longus
   - Flexor digitorum longus
   - Posterior tibialis
   - Extensor hallicus longus
   - Extensor digitorum longus
   - Peroneus longus

   - Peroneus brevis
   - Peroneus tertius
   - Gastrocnemius
   - Soleus

5. Demonstrate, on someone other than yourself, functional tests to determine the normalcy of each of the muscles and ligaments in Competencies 3 and 4. Use tests to determine the stability of the ligaments listed in Competency 3 and the flexibility and strength of the muscles listed in Competency 4.

6. Using surface anatomy, palpate or draw, on someone other than yourself, the course of each of the following nerves:

   - Anterior tibial
   - Posterior tibial
   - Peroneal

Use the following list of injuries to complete Competencies 7 through 11.

> First-degree ankle sprain
> Second-degree ankle sprain
> Third-degree ankle sprain
> Sprain-dislocation
> Ankle sprain
> Fractures
> Stress fractures
> Avulsion fractures

7. Explain and demonstrate the mechanisms by which each of the listed injuries occurs. Name the three sports in which each injury is most likely to occur, and explain any differences among the injury occurrences/mechanisms in those sports.

8. Explain and demonstrate, on someone other than yourself, the appropriate immediate care procedures for each listed injury. Explain the objectives, and criteria for progression, for each step in the procedure.

9. Demonstrate, on someone other than yourself, a complete rehabilitation program for each listed injury. As you proceed, explain the objectives and procedures of each step in the program. Explain the measurement criteria for advancing from one step to another.
10. Using pictures or illustrations, explain the objectives and procedures of prophylactic taping, padding, or bandaging for the listed injuries as appropriate.

11. Demonstrate or explain procedures for preventing each listed injury.

Mastery and Demonstration

Master these skills through study, consultation with a Level 3 student, and practice on your own and with other Level 2 students. Then demonstrate your competence to a faculty member or a Level 3 student.

Practice

	Date	Partner		Comments
1.	_____	_____		
2.	_____	_____		

Grade _____ Date _____ Approved by _____
Comments:

Lower Leg Injury Management

Competencies

1. Name and palpate each of the following bones and any prominent features listed:

   - Tibia
       Medial condyle
       Lateral condyle
       Gerdy's tubercle
       Patellar tubercle
       Malleolus
   - Fibula
       Head
       Malleolus

2. On someone other than yourself, palpate or draw the joint line, then perform active and passive joint range of motion tests, and tests to determine joint stability for each of the following articulations:

   - Proximal tibiofibular
   - Distal tibiofibular

3. Using surface anatomy, draw or palpate, on someone other than yourself, the origins and course of interosseous ligament.

4. Using surface anatomy, draw or palpate, on someone other than yourself, the origin, insertion, and course of each of the following muscles. Then tell the major function of the muscle.

   - Anterior tibialis
   - Posterior tibialis
   - Flexor hallicus longus
   - Flexor digitorum longus
   - Extensor hallicus longus
   - Extensor digitorum longus
   - Peroneus longus
   - Peroneus brevis
   - Peroneus tertius
   - Gastrocnemius
   - Soleus

5. Demonstrate, on someone other than yourself, functional tests to determine the normalcy of each of the muscles and ligaments

in Competencies 3 and 4. Use tests to determine the stability of the ligament listed in Competency 3 and the flexibility and strength of the muscles listed in Competency 4.

6. Using surface anatomy, palpate or draw, on someone other than yourself, each of the following structures:

   - Common peroneal nerve (entire course)
   - Pedal pulse

Use the following list of injuries to complete Competencies 7 through 11.

   Achilles tendon strain

   Achilles bursitis and tenosynovitis

   Anterior shin splints

   Posterior shin splints

   Anterior compartment syndrome

   Muscular strains and ruptures

   Contusions

   Peroneal nerve contusion

   Fractures

   Stress fractures

7. Explain and demonstrate the mechanisms by which each of the listed injuries occurs. Name the three sports in which the injury is most likely to occur, and explain any differences among the injury occurrences/mechanisms in those sports.

8. Explain and demonstrate, on someone other than yourself, the appropriate immediate care procedures for each listed injury. Explain the objectives, and criteria for progression, for each step in the procedure.

9. Demonstrate, on someone other than yourself, a complete rehabilitation program for each listed injury. As you proceed, explain the objectives and procedures of each step in the program. Explain the measurement criteria for advancing from one step to another.

10. Using pictures or illustrations, explain the objectives and procedures of prophylactic taping, padding, or bandaging for the listed injuries as appropriate.
11. Demonstrate or explain procedures for preventing each listed injury.

Mastery and Demonstration

Master these skills through study, consultation with a Level 3 student, and practice on your own and with other Level 2 students. Then demonstrate your competence to a faculty member or a Level 3 student.

Practice

	Date	Partner	Comments
1.	_____	_____	
2.	_____	_____	

Grade _____ Date _____ Approved by _____

Comments:

Knee Injury Management

Competencies

1. Name and palpate each of the following bones and any prominent features listed:
   - Femur
     Condyles
     Epicondyles
   - Tibia
     Medial condyle
     Lateral condyle
     Gerdy's tubercle
   - Fibula
     Head
   - Patella

2. On someone other than yourself, palpate or draw the joint line, then perform active and passive joint range of motion tests, and tests to determine joint stability for each of the following articulations:
   - Medial tibiofemoral joint
   - Lateral tibiofemoral joint
   - Patellotibial joint

3. Using surface anatomy, draw or palpate, on someone other than yourself, the origins and course of each of the following ligaments:
   - Lateral capsular
   - Lateral collateral
   - Medial capsular (deep collateral)
     Posterior fibers
     Middle fibers
     Anterior fibers
   - Medial collateral (superficial collateral)
   - Anterior cruciate
   - Posterior cruciate
   - Patellar

4. Using surface anatomy, draw or palpate, on someone other than yourself, the origin, insertion, and course of each of the following muscles. Then tell the major function of the muscle.
   - Biceps femoris (long and short heads)
   - Semitendinosus
   - Semimembranosis
   - Rectus femoris
   - Vastus medialis
   - Vastus intermedius
   - Vastus lateralis
   - Sartorius
   - Tensor fasciae latae
   - Iliotibial band
   - Gracilis
   - Gastrocnemius (medial and lateral heads)
   - Popliteus

5. Demonstrate, on someone other than yourself, functional tests to determine the normalcy of each of the muscles and ligaments in Competencies 3 and 4. Use tests to determine the stability of the ligaments listed in Competency 3 and the flexibility and strength of the muscles listed in Competency 4.

6. Using surface anatomy, palpate or draw, on someone other than yourself, the location or course of each of the following structures:
   - Common peroneal nerve
   - Suprapatellar bursa
   - Patellar bursa
   - Infrapatellar fat pad
   - Infrapatellar bursa
   - Superficial bursa

Use the following list of injuries to complete Competencies 7 through 11.

Torn medial meniscus

Torn lateral meniscus

Anterior cruciate sprain

Posterior cruciate sprain

Medial collateral (superficial) sprain

Medial collateral (deep) sprain

Lateral collateral sprain

Anteriomedial rotary instability

Anteriolateral rotary instability

Bursitis

Capsular contusion

Contused vastus medialis

Patellofemoral joint pain

Patellar tendinitis

Fractured patella

Baker's cyst

Synovial plica

Hyperextended knee

Osgood-Schlatter disease

Iliotibial band syndrome

Distal hamstring strain

7. Explain and demonstrate the mechanisms by which each of the listed injuries occurs. Name the three sports in which the injury is most likely to occur, and explain any differences among the injury occurrences/mechanisms in those sports.

8. Explain and demonstrate, on someone other than yourself, the appropriate immediate care procedures for each listed injury. Explain the objectives, and criteria for progressing, for each step in the procedure.

9. Demonstrate, on someone other than yourself, a complete rehabilitation program for each listed injury. As you proceed, explain the objectives and procedures of each step in the program. Explain the measurement criteria for advancing from one step to another.

10. Using pictures or illustrations, explain the objectives and procedures of prophylactic taping, padding, or bandaging for the listed injuries as appropriate.

11. Demonstrate or explain procedures for preventing each listed injury.

Mastery and Demonstration

Master these skills through study, consultation with a Level 3 student, and practice on your own and with other Level 2 students. Then demonstrate your competence to a faculty member or a Level 3 student.

Practice

	Date	Partner	Comments
1.	_____	_____	
2.	_____	_____	

Grade _____ Date _____ Approved by _____

Comments:

Thigh Injury Management

Competencies

1. Name and palpate each of the following bones and any prominent features listed:
   - Femur
     Condyles
     Epicondyles
   - Tibia
     Medial condyle
     Lateral condyle
     Gerdy's tubercle
     Patellar tubercle
   - Fibula
     Head
   - Patella

2. On someone other than yourself, palpate or draw the joint line, then perform active and passive joint range of motion tests, and tests to determine joint stability for each of the following articulations:
   - Medial tibiofemoral
   - Lateral tibiofemoral
   - Patellotibial

3. Using surface anatomy, draw or palpate, on someone other than yourself, the origin, insertion, and course of each of the following muscles. Then tell the major function of the muscle.
   - Biceps femoris (long and short heads)
   - Semitendinosus
   - Semimembranosis
   - Rectus femoris
   - Vastus medialis
   - Vastus intermedius
   - Vastus lateralis
   - Sartorius
   - Tensor fasciae latae
   - Iliotibial band
   - Gracilis

4. Demonstrate, on someone other than yourself, functional tests to determine the normalcy of each of the muscles in Competency 3. Use tests to determine the flexibility and strength of those muscles.

5. Using surface anatomy, palpate or draw, on someone other than yourself, the course of each of the following nerves:
   - Femoral
   - Sciatic

Use the following list of injuries to complete Competencies 6 through 10.

Quadriceps contusion

Quadriceps strain

Hamstring strain

Femoral fracture

Myositis ossificans

Patellar tendon rupture

6. Explain and demonstrate the mechanisms by which each of the listed injuries occurs. Name the three sports in which the injury is most likely to occur, and explain any differences among the injury occurrences/mechanisms in those sports.

7. Explain and demonstrate, on someone other than yourself, the appropriate immediate care procedures for each listed injury. Explain the purpose, goals and objectives, and criteria for progression, for each step in the procedure.

8. Demonstrate, on someone other than yourself, a complete rehabilitation program for each listed injury. As you proceed, explain the objectives and procedures of each step in the program. Explain the measurement criteria for advancing from one step to another.

9. Using pictures or illustrations, explain the objectives and procedures of prophylactic taping, padding, or bandaging for the listed injuries as appropriate.

10. Demonstrate or explain procedures for preventing each listed injury.

Mastery and Demonstration

Master these skills through study, consultation with a Level 3 student, and practice on your own and with other Level 2 students. Then demonstrate your competence to a faculty member or a Level 3 student.

Practice

	Date	Partner	Comments
1.	_____	_____	
2.	_____	_____	

Grade _____ Date _____ Approved by _____

Comments:

Hip and Groin Injury Management

Competencies

1. Name and palpate each of the following bones and any prominent features listed:

   - Ilium
     Crest
     Tubercle
     Anterior inferior spine
     Anterior superior spine
     Posterior superior spine
   - Pubis
     Ramus
     Tubercle
   - Ischium
     Tubercle or tuberosity
   - Femur
     Greater trochanter
     Lesser trochanter
     Linea aspera
   - Spine
     Lumbar vertebra
     Sacrum
     Coccyx

2. On someone other than yourself, palpate or draw the joint line, then perform active and passive joint range of motion tests, and tests to determine joint stability for each of the following articulations:

   - Sacroiliac
   - Lumbosacral
   - Hip

3. Using surface anatomy, palpate or draw, on someone other than yourself, the origins and course of each of the following ligaments:

   - Inguinal
   - Supraspinous
   - Interspinous
   - Intertransverse
   - Longitudinal (posterior and anterior)

4. Using surface anatomy, palpate or draw, on someone other than yourself, the origin, insertion, and course of each of the following muscles and tendons. Then tell the major function of the muscle or tendon.

   - Gluteus maximus
   - Gluteus medius
   - Gluteus minimus
   - Tensor fasciae latae
   - Iliotibial band
   - Biceps femoris (long and short heads)
   - Semitendinosus
   - Semimembranosis
   - Iliopsoas
   - Psoas major
   - Iliacus
   - Rectus femoris
   - Sartorius
   - Gracilis
   - Adductor longus
   - Adductor brevis
   - Adductor magnus
   - Latissimus dorsi
   - Paraspinal
   - External obliques
   - Internal obliques
   - Transverse abdominis

5. Demonstrate, on someone other than yourself, functional tests to determine the normalcy of each of the muscles and ligaments in Competencies 3 and 4. Use tests to determine the stability of the ligaments listed in Competency 3 and the flexibility and strength of the muscles listed in Competency 4.

6. Using surface anatomy, palpate or draw, on someone other than yourself, the location or course of each of the following structures:

   - Sciatic nerve
   - Lateral cutaneous nerve
   - Trochanteric bursae
   - Iliopsoas bursae

Use the following list of injuries to complete Competencies 7 through 11.

Snapping hip

Lateral hip pain

Hip sprain

Hip pointer

Dislocated hip

Proximal hamstring strain

Proximal sartorius strain

Hip flexor strain

Groin strain

Gluteal strain

Hernia

Contused genitalia

Spermatic cord torsion

Traumatic hydrocele of the tunica vaginalis

Femur fracture

Pelvic fracture

Trochanteric bursitis

Iliopsoas bursitis

7. Explain and demonstrate the mechanisms by which each of the listed injuries occurs. Name the three sports in which the injury is most likely to occur, and explain any differences among the injury occurrences/mechanisms in those sports.

8. Explain and demonstrate, on someone other than yourself, the appropriate immediate care procedures for each listed injury. Explain the objectives, and criteria for progression, for each step in the procedure.

9. Demonstrate, on someone other than yourself, a complete rehabilitation program for each listed injury. As you proceed, explain the objectives and procedures of each step in the program. Explain the measurement criteria for advancing from one step to another.

10. Using pictures or illustrations, explain the objectives and procedures of prophylactic taping, padding, or bandaging for the listed injuries as appropriate.

11. Demonstrate or explain procedures for preventing each listed injury.

Mastery and Demonstration

Master these skills through study, consultation with a Level 3 student, and practice on your own and with other Level 2 students. Then demonstrate your competence to a faculty member or a Level 3 student.

Practice

    Date   Partner   Comments

1. _____ _____

2. _____ _____

Grade _____ Date _____ Approved by _____

Comments:

Low Back Injury Management

Competencies

1. Name and palpate each of the following bones and any prominent features listed:

   - Ilium
     Crest
     Tubercle
     Anterior inferior spine
     Anterior superior spine
     Posterior superior spine
   - Pubis
     Tubercle
   - Ischium
     Tubercle or tuberosity
   - Femur
     Greater trochanter
   - Spine
     Lumbar vertebrae
     Spinous processes
     Sacrum
     Coccyx

2. On someone other than yourself, palpate or draw the joint line, then perform active and passive joint range of motion tests, and tests to determine joint stability for each of the following articulations:

   - Sacroiliac
   - Lumbosacral
   - Hip

3. Using surface anatomy, palpate or draw, on someone other than yourself, the origins and course of each of the following ligaments:

   - Supraspinous
   - Interspinous
   - Intertransverse
   - Longitudinal (posterior and anterior)

4. Using surface anatomy, palpate or draw, on someone other than yourself, the origin, insertion, and course of each of the following muscles. Then tell the major function of the muscle.

   - Rectus abdominis
   - External oblique
   - Internal oblique
   - Transverse abdominis
   - Gluteus maximus
   - Gluteus medius
   - Gluteus minimus
   - Tensor fasciae latae
   - Hamstrings
   - Iliopsoas
   - Psoas major
   - Iliacus
   - Paraspinal

5. Demonstrate, on someone other than yourself, functional tests to determine the normalcy of each of the muscles and ligaments in Competencies 3 and 4. Use tests to determine the stability of the ligaments listed in Competency 3 and the flexibility and strength of the muscles listed in Competency 4.

6. Using surface anatomy, palpate or draw, on someone other than yourself, the location of each of the following organs:

   - Bladder
   - Liver
   - Spleen
   - Kidneys

Use the following list of injuries to complete Competencies 7 through 11.

Lumbar sprain/strain

Lumbar contusion

Lumbosacral sprain/strain

Sacroiliac sprain

Disc rupture

Sciatica

Spondylolysis

Spondylolisthesis

Spondylitis

Transverse spinous process fracture

7. Explain and demonstrate the mechanisms by which each of the listed injuries occurs.

Name the three sports in which each injury is most likely to occur, and explain any differences among the injury occurrences/mechanisms in those sports.

8. Explain and demonstrate, on someone other than yourself, the appropriate immediate care procedures for each listed injury. Explain the objectives, and criteria for progression, for each step in the procedure.

9. Demonstrate, on someone other than yourself, a complete rehabilitation program for each listed injury. As you proceed, explain the purpose, goals and objectives, and procedures of each step in the program. Explain the measurement criteria for advancing from one step to another.

10. Using pictures or illustrations, explain the objectives and procedures of prophylactic taping, padding, or bandaging for the listed injuries as appropriate.

11. Demonstrate or explain procedures for preventing each listed injury.

Mastery and Demonstration

Master these skills through study, consultation with a Level 3 student, and practice on your own and with other Level 2 students. Then demonstrate your competence to a faculty member or a Level 3 student.

Practice

Date   Partner   Comments

1. _____   _____

2. _____   _____

Grade _____ Date _____ Approved by _____

Comments:

Chest and Abdominal Injury Management

Competencies

1. Name and palpate each of the following bones and any prominent features listed:
   - Ilium
     Crest
     Tubercle
     Anterior inferior spine
     Anterior superior spine
     Posterior superior spine
   - Spine
     Thoracic vertebrae
     Spinous processes
   - Rib cage
     Ribs
     Floating ribs
     Costal cartilage
   - Sternum
     Manubrium
     Body
     Xiphoid process

2. On someone other than yourself, palpate or draw the joint line, then perform active and passive joint range of motion tests, and tests to determine joint stability for each of the following articulations:
   - Sternoclavicular
   - Costosternal
   - Costovertebral
   - Costochondral

3. Using surface anatomy, draw or palpate, on someone other than yourself, the location of each of the following internal organs:
   - Heart
   - Lungs
   - Pancreas
   - Liver
   - Spleen
   - Kidney
   - Stomach
   - Intestine
   - Gallbladder
   - Urinary bladder

4. Using surface anatomy, draw or palpate, on someone other than yourself, the origin, insertion, and course of each of the following muscles. Then tell what the major function of the muscle is.
   - Rectus abdominis
   - Obliques
   - Transverse abdominis
   - Latissimus dorsi
   - Erector spinae
   - Quadratus lumborum
   - Intercostals
   - Diaphragm

5. Demonstrate, on someone other than yourself, functional tests to determine the normalcy of each of the muscles and organs in Competencies 3 and 4. Use tests to determine the stability of the organs listed in Competency 3 and the flexibility and strength of the muscles listed in Competency 4.

6. Using surface anatomy, palpate or draw, on someone other than yourself, the course of the phrenic nerves.

Use the following list of injuries to complete Competencies 7 through 11.

Abdominal muscular strain

Rectus abdominis contusion

Spleen rupture

Kidney contusion

Stitch in the side

Wind knocked out

Sternoclavicular (S-C) separation

Sternal fracture

Rib fracture

Rib contusion

Costochondral dislocation

Pneumothorax

Hemothorax

7. Explain and demonstrate the mechanisms by which each of the listed injuries occurs. Name the three sports in which each injury is most likely to occur, and explain any differences among the injury occurrences/mechanisms in those sports.

8. Explain and demonstrate, on someone other than yourself, the appropriate immediate care procedures for each listed injury. Explain the objectives, and criteria for progression, for each step in the procedure.

9. Demonstrate, on someone other than yourself, a complete rehabilitation program for each listed injury. As you proceed, explain the objectives and procedures of each step in the program. Explain the measurement criteria for advancing from one step to another.

10. Using pictures or illustrations, explain the objectives and procedures of prophylactic taping, padding, or bandaging for the listed injuries as appropriate.

11. Demonstrate or explain procedures for preventing each listed injury.

Mastery and Demonstration

Master these skills through study, consultation with a Level 3 student, and practice on your own and with other Level 2 students. Then demonstrate your competence to a faculty member or a Level 3 student.

Practice

	Date	Partner	Comments
1.	_____	_____	
2.	_____	_____	

Grade _____ Date _____ Approved by _____

Comments:

Shoulder Injury Management

Competencies

1. Name and palpate each of the following bones and any prominent features listed:
   - Ribs
   - Sternum
     Manubrium
     Body
   - Clavicle
   - Scapula
     Suprapatellar fossa
     Spine
     Infrapatellar fossa
     Acromium process
     Coracoid process
   - Humerus
     Greater trochanter
     Lesser trochanter
     Bicipital groove

2. On someone other than yourself, palpate or draw the joint line, then perform active and passive joint range of motion tests, and tests to determine joint stability for each of the following articulations:
   - Glenohumeral
   - Acromioclavicular
   - Coracoclavicular
   - Sternoclavicular

3. Using surface anatomy, draw or palpate, on someone other than yourself, the origins and course of each of the following ligaments or bursa:
   - Glenohumeral
     Anterior
     Middle
     Posterior
   - Acromioclavicular
   - Coracoclavicular
   - Coracoacromial
   - Sternoclavicular
   - Subacromial bursa
   - Subdeltoid bursa

4. Using surface anatomy, draw or palpate, on someone other than yourself, the origin, insertion, and course of each of the following muscles. Then tell what the major function of the muscle is.
   - Biceps (both heads)
   - Triceps (all three heads)
   - Deltoid (all three portions)
   - Pectoralis major
   - Pectoralis minor
   - Teres major
   - Teres minor
   - Latissimus dorsi
   - Supraspinatus
   - Infraspinatus
   - Subscapularis
   - Trapezius
   - Rhomboids
   - Levator scapulae
   - Serratus anterior
   - Subclavius

5. Demonstrate, on someone other than yourself, functional tests to determine the normalcy of each of the muscles and ligaments in Competencies 3 and 4. Use tests to determine the stability of the ligaments listed in Competency 3 and the flexibility and strength of the muscles listed in Competency 4.

6. Using surface anatomy, palpate or draw, on someone other than yourself, the course of each of the following nerves:
   - Brachial plexus
   - Axillary nerve

Use the following list of injuries to complete Competencies 7 through 11.

Sternoclavicular sprain/dislocation

Clavicular fracture

Acromioclavicular contusion

Acromioclavicular sprain

Glenohumeral dislocation

Recurrent glenohumeral dislocation

Rotator cuff impingement

Rotator cuff strain

Subacromial bursitis

Bicipital tenosynovitis

Bicipital subluxation

Thoracic outlet syndrome

Epiphyseal fracture

Throwing injuries

7. Explain and demonstrate the mechanisms by which each of the listed injuries occurs. Name the three sports in which each injury is most likely to occur, and explain any differences among the injury occurrences/mechanisms in those sports.

8. Explain and demonstrate, on someone other than yourself, the appropriate immediate care procedures for each listed injury. Explain the objectives, and criteria for progression, for each step in the procedure.

9. Demonstrate, on someone other than yourself, a complete rehabilitation program for each listed injury. As you proceed, explain the objectives and procedures of each step in the program. Explain the measurement criteria for advancing from one step to another.

10. Using pictures or illustrations, explain the objectives and procedures of prophylactic taping, padding, or bandaging for the listed injuries as appropriate.

11. Demonstrate or explain procedures for preventing each listed injury.

Mastery and Demonstration

Master these skills through study, consultation with a Level 3 student, and practice on your own and with other Level 2 students. Then demonstrate your competence to a faculty member or a Level 3 student.

Practice

	Date	Partner	Comments
1.	_____	_____	
2.	_____	_____	

Grade _____ Date _____ Approved by _____

Comments:

Arm and Elbow Injury Management

Competencies

1. Name and palpate each of the following bones and any prominent features listed:

   - Humerus
     Greater trochanter
     Lesser trochanter
     Bicipital groove
     Capitulum
     Olecranon fossa
   - Ulna
     Olecranon process
     Coronoid process
     Trochlea notch
     Radial notch
     Interosseous border
   - Radius
     Head
     Interosseous border
     Ulnar notch

2. On someone other than yourself, palpate or draw the joint line, then perform active and passive joint range of motion tests, and tests to determine joint stability for each of the following articulations:

   - Radiohumeral
   - Ulnahumeral
   - Proximal radioulnar

3. Using surface anatomy, draw or palpate, on someone other than yourself, the origins and course of each of the following ligaments or bursa:

   - Anular
   - Ulnar collateral
   - Radial collateral
   - Interosseous
   - Olecranon bursa
   - Radiohumeral bursa

4. Using surface anatomy, draw or palpate, on someone other than yourself, the origin, insertion, and course of each of the following muscles. Then tell what the major function of the muscle is.

   - Biceps (both heads)
   - Triceps (all three heads)
   - Coracobrachialis
   - Brachialis
   - Brachioradialis
   - Anconeus
   - Pronator teres
   - Pronator quadratus
   - Flexor carpi radialis
   - Flexor carpi ulnaris
   - Extensor carpi radialis
   - Extensor carpi ulnaris
   - Extensor digitorum
   - Supinator

5. Demonstrate, on someone other than yourself, functional tests to determine the normalcy of each of the muscles and ligaments in Competencies 3 and 4. Use tests to determine the stability of the ligaments listed in Competency 3 and the flexibility and strength of the muscles listed in Competency 4.

6. Using surface anatomy, palpate on someone other than yourself each of the following structures:

   - Median nerve
   - Radial nerve
   - Ulnar nerve
   - Radial pulse

Use the following list of injuries to complete Competencies 7 through 11.

Bicipital strain

Humoral fracture

Epiphyseal fracture

Humeral contusion

Humeral exostoses

Supracondylar fracture

Olecranon bursitis

Medial elbow strain

Medial collateral ligament sprain

Elbow hyperextension

Elbow dislocation

Elbow fractures

Radial nerve injury

Throwing injuries

Epicondylitis humeri

Forearm contusion

Radial head fracture

Forearm splints

7. Explain and demonstrate the mechanisms by which each of the listed injuries occurs. Name the three sports in which each injury is most likely to occur, and explain any differences among the injury occurrences/ mechanisms in those sports.

8. Explain and demonstrate, on someone other than yourself, the appropriate immediate care procedures for each listed injury. Explain the objectives, and criteria for progression, for each step in the procedure.

9. Demonstrate, on someone other than yourself, a complete rehabilitation program for each listed injury. As you proceed, explain the objectives and procedures of each step in the program. Explain the measurement criteria for advancing from one step to another.

10. Using pictures or illustrations, explain the objectives and procedures of prophylactic taping, padding, or bandaging for the listed injuries as appropriate.

11. Demonstrate or explain procedures for preventing each listed injury.

Mastery and Demonstration

Master these skills through study, consultation with a Level 3 student, and practice on your own and with other Level 2 students. Then demonstrate your competence to a faculty member or a Level 3 student.

Practice

	Date	Partner	Comments
1.	_____	_____	
2.	_____	_____	

Grade _____ Date _____ Approved by _____

Comments:

Wrist and Hand Injury Management

Competencies

1. Name and palpate each of the following bones and any prominent features listed:
   - Ulna
     - Styloid process
   - Radius
     - Styloid process
   - Pisiform
   - Triquetrum
   - Lunate
   - Scaphoid
   - Hamate
   - Capitate
   - Trapezoid
   - Trapezium
   - Metacarpals
   - Phalanges
     - Proximal
     - Middle
     - Distal

2. On someone other than yourself, palpate or draw the joint line, then perform active and passive joint range of motion tests, and tests to determine joint stability for each of the following articulations:
   - Inferior radial-ulnar
   - Radial-carpal
   - Ulnar-carpal
   - Mid-carpal
   - Carpal-metacarpal
   - Proximal interphangeal
   - Distal interphangeal

3. Using surface anatomy, draw or palpate, on someone other than yourself, the origins and course of each of the following ligaments:
   - Flexor retinaculum
   - Ulnar collateral
   - Radial collateral
   - PIP and DIP collateral
   - Palmer
   - Deep transverse

4. Using surface anatomy, draw or palpate, on someone other than yourself, the origin, insertion, and course of each of the following muscles. Then tell what the major function of the muscle is.
   - Palmaris longis
   - Extensor pollicis longis
   - Flexor carpi radialis
   - Flexor carpi ulnaris
   - Brachioradialis
   - Extensor carpi radialis
   - Extensor carpi ulnaris
   - Extensor digitorum
   - Thenar
   - Hypothenar
   - Lumbricles
   - Palmer interossei
   - Dorsal interossei

5. Demonstrate, on someone other than yourself, functional tests to determine the normalcy of each of the muscles and ligaments in Competencies 3 and 4. Use tests to determine the stability of the ligaments listed in Competency 3 and the flexibility and strength of the muscles listed in Competency 4.

6. Using surface anatomy, palpate, on someone other than yourself, each of the following structures:
   - Median nerve
   - Radial nerve
   - Ulnar nerve
   - Radial pulse

Use the following list of injuries to complete Competencies 7 through 11.

Colles' fracture

Carpal navicular fracture

Lunate dislocation

Hamate fracture

Radio-ulnar sprain

Wrist ganglion

Carpal sprain

Carpal tunnel syndrome

Hand contusion

Thumb ulnar collateral ligament sprain

PIP sprain

Boutonniere deformity

Interphangeal dislocations

Metacarpal fractures

Phangeal fractures

Mallet finger

Subungual hematoma

7. Explain and demonstrate the mechanisms by which each of the listed injuries occurs. Name the three sports in which each injury is most likely to occur, and explain any differences among the injury occurrences/ mechanisms in those sports.

8. Explain and demonstrate, on someone other than yourself, the appropriate immediate care procedures for each listed injury. Explain the objectives, and criteria for progression, for each step in the procedure.

9. Demonstrate, on someone other than yourself, a complete rehabilitation program for each listed injury. As you proceed, explain the objectives and procedures of each step in the program. Explain the measurement criteria for advancing from one step to another.

10. Using pictures or illustrations, explain the objectives and procedures of prophylactic taping, padding, or bandaging for the listed injuries as appropriate.

11. Demonstrate or explain procedures for preventing each listed injury.

Mastery and Demonstration

Master these skills through study, consultation with a Level 3 student, and practice on your own and with other Level 2 students. Then demonstrate your competence to a faculty member or a Level 3 student.

Practice

Date   Partner   Comments

1. _____   _____

2. _____   _____

Grade _____ Date _____ Approved by _____

Comments:

Head and Neck Injury Management

Competencies

1. Name and palpate each of the following bones and any prominent features listed:
   - Skull
     Parietal
     Occipital
   - Cervical vertebra
     Spinous processes
     Transverse processes
   - Mastoid process
   - Atlas
   - Axis
   - Clavicle
   - First rib

2. On someone other than yourself, palpate or draw the joint line, then perform active and passive joint range of motion tests, and tests to determine joint stability for the cervical intervertebral articulation.

3. Using surface anatomy, draw or palpate, on someone other than yourself, the origins and course of each of the following ligaments:
   - Nuchal
   - Ligamentum flavum
   - Ligamentum nuchae

4. Using surface anatomy, draw or palpate, on someone other than yourself, the origin, insertion, and course of each of the following muscles. Then tell what the major function of the muscle is.
   - Sternocleidomastoid
   - Scalene (three portions)
   - Trapezius
   - Posterior vertebral

5. Demonstrate, on someone other than yourself, functional tests to determine the normalcy of each of the muscles and ligaments in Competencies 3 and 4. Use tests to determine the stability of the ligaments listed in Competency 3 and the flexibility and strength of the muscles listed in Competency 4.

6. Using surface anatomy, palpate or draw, on someone other than yourself, the location of each of the following anatomical structures:
   - Brachial plexus
   - Myotomes
   - Dermatomes

Use the following list of injuries to complete Competencies 7 through 10.

Skull fracture

Concussion

Intracranial bleeding

Cervical fracture

Cervical dislocation

Cervical sprains

Cervical strains

Neck contusion

Neck burner

7. Explain and demonstrate the mechanisms by which each of the listed injuries occurs. Name the three sports in which each injury is most likely to occur, and explain any differences among the injury occurrences/mechanisms in those sports.

8. Explain and demonstrate, on someone other than yourself, the appropriate immediate care procedures for each listed injury. Explain the objectives, and criteria for progression, for each step in the procedure.

9. Demonstrate, on someone other than yourself, a complete rehabilitation program for each listed injury. As you proceed, explain the objectives and procedures of each step in the program. Explain the measurement criteria for advancing from one step to another.

10. Demonstrate or explain procedures for preventing the listed injuries as appropriate.

Mastery and Demonstration

Master these skills through study, consultation with a Level 3 student, and practice on your own and with other Level 2 students. Then demonstrate your competence to a faculty member or a Level 3 student.

Practice

     Date   Partner   Comments

1. _____ _____

2. _____ _____

Grade _____ Date _____ Approved by _____

Comments:

Facial Injury Management

Competencies

1. Name and palpate each of the following bones and any prominent features listed:
   - Mandible
   - Maxilla
   - Mastoid process
   - Nasal (both)
   - Skull
     Frontal
     Temporal
   - Temporomandibular
2. On someone other than yourself, palpate or draw the joint line, then perform active and passive joint range of motion tests, and tests to determine joint stability for the temporomandibular joint.
3. Identify the location of each of the following anatomical structures:
   - Nasal passages
   - Auris
   - Eye
     Cornea
     Lens
     Iris
     Chamber
     Retina

Use the following list of injuries to complete Competencies 4 through 8.

Scalp hematoma

Lacerations

Jaw fracture

Jaw dislocation

Dental injuries

Foreign body in the eye

Contact lens lost in the eye

Corneal abrasions

Lens or iris injury

Eye chamber hemorrhage

Detached retina

Nose bleed

Nasal fracture

Hematoma auris

Ruptured eardrum

Swimmer's ear

Foreign body in the ear

4. Explain and demonstrate the mechanisms by which each of the listed injuries occurs. Name the three sports in which each injury is most likely to occur, and explain any differences among the injury occurrences/mechanisms in those sports.
5. Explain and demonstrate, on someone other than yourself, the appropriate immediate care procedures for each listed injury. Explain the objectives, and criteria for progression, for each step in the procedure.
6. Demonstrate, on someone other than yourself, a complete rehabilitation program for each listed injury. As you proceed, explain the objectives and procedures of each step in the program. Explain the measurement criteria for advancing from one step to another.
7. Using pictures or illustrations, explain the objectives and procedures of prophylactic taping, padding, or bandaging for the listed injuries as appropriate.
8. Demonstrate or explain procedures for preventing each listed injury.

Mastery and Demonstration

Master these skills through study, consultation with a Level 3 student, and practice on your own and with other Level 2 students. Then demonstrate your competence to a faculty member or a Level 3 student.

Practice

     Date   Partner   Comments

1. _____ _____

2. _____ _____

Grade _____ Date _____ Approved by _____

Comments:

Management of Dermatological Conditions

Competencies

1. Describe, with the use of pictures, the structure of the skin (including all the layers).

Use the following list of conditions to complete Competencies 2 through 4.

Blisters

Common fungal infections

Common bacterial infections

Herpes simplex

Herpes zoster

Impetigo

Cellulitis

Urticaria

Nonspecific dermatitis

Common infestations

2. Explain and demonstrate the mechanisms by which each of the listed conditions occurs.

Except for herpes, which is not more common in one sport than in another, name the three sports in which each condition is most likely to occur, and explain any differences among the injury occurrences/mechanisms in those sports.

3. Explain and demonstrate, on someone other than yourself, the appropriate management procedures for each listed condition. Explain the objectives, and criteria for progression, for each step in the procedure.

4. Demonstrate or explain procedures for preventing each listed condition.

Mastery and Demonstration

Master these skills through study, consultation with a Level 3 student, and practice on your own and with other Level 2 students. Then demonstrate your competence to a faculty member or a Level 3 student.

Practice

Date   Partner   Comments

1. _____ _____

2. _____ _____

Grade _____ Date _____ Approved by _____

Comments:

Management of Common Illnesses

Competencies

Use the following list of conditions to complete Competencies 1 through 4.

Colds
Streptococcal infections
Infectious mononucleosis
Canker sores
Sinusitis
Bronchitis
Pneumonia
Hypertension
Urine abnormalities
Menstrual irregularities
Common venereal diseases
Allergies
Asthma
Diarrhea
Constipation
Hemorrhoids
Appendicitis
Indigestion
Diabetes
Epilepsy

Insect stings
Shock
Heat illnesses

1. Explain and demonstrate the mechanisms by which each of the listed conditions develop. Tell how each condition affects athletes' performances in football, basketball, baseball/softball, track and field, and two other sports.
2. Explain and demonstrate, where appropriate, on someone other than yourself, the appropriate management procedures for each listed condition. Explain the objectives, and criteria for progression, for each step in the procedure.
3. Explain guidelines for participation (practice and games) for athletes with each of the listed conditions.
4. Demonstrate or explain procedures for preventing each listed condition.

Mastery and Demonstration

Master these skills through study, consultation with a Level 3 student, and practice on your own and with other Level 2 students. Then demonstrate your competence to a faculty member or a Level 3 student.

Module G15—Management of Common Illnesses (Continued)

Practice

	Date	Partner	Comments
1.	_____	_____	
2.	_____	_____	

Grade _____ Date _____ Approved by _____

Comments:

Oral/Practical Examination

Competencies

1. Complete your program's oral/practical examination with a score of 85% or better.

Date taken _____ Score _____ Approved by _____

Reexamination _____ Score _____ Approved by _____

Level 3

Team Trainer

Competencies

1. Serve as a team trainer with an athletic team during their entire sport season (preseason conditioning through off-season conditioning). Among other things, do the following:

   a. Perform physical examination of athletes.
   b. Test team's level of conditioning.

   c. Inspect training room for compliance with safety and sanitary standards.
   d. Be a team leader in a mock removal from the field or court of an athlete with a possible cervical injury.
   e. Inventory equipment and supplies.
   f. Prepare an equipment and supply purchase request for next season, based on your inventory.

Grade _____ Date _____ Approved by _____

Comments:

Internship (Field Experience)

Competencies

1. Serve as a team trainer with either a high school for one semester or an athletic team at your university during their entire sport season, including preseason conditioning, regular season, and off-season conditioning. (Note: This must be in addition to and following Module X10.)

Grade _____ Date _____ Approved by _____

Comments:

Student Athletic Training Supervision

Competencies

1. Work with at least five different Level 1 and Level 2 students on a total of 20 modules. This includes reviewing material with them and testing them for their mastery of the material. Most of this experience should be with Level 2 students.

Date	Person examined	Module	Grade given
1.			
2.			
3.			
4.			
5.			
6.			
7.			
8.			
9.			
10.			
11.			
12.			
13.			
14.			
15.			
16.			
17.			
18.			
19.			
20.			

Grade _____ Date _____ Approved by _____

Comments:

Administration of Oral/Practical Examination

Competencies

1. Serve as an examiner for at least five different oral/practical examinations.

	Person examined	*Date*
1.	_____	_____
2.	_____	_____
3.	_____	_____
4.	_____	_____
5.	_____	_____
6.	_____	_____
7.	_____	_____
8.	_____	_____

Grade _____ Date _____ Approved by _____

Comments:

Study Aids

Recommended Resources

Most of the following references are recommended by the NATA for use in working toward NATA certification. Some of these have been selected to be cross-referenced with this text (see pp. 94-102).

1. American Academy of Ophthalmology: *The Athlete's Eye.* San Francisco: AAO, 1982.
2. American Academy of Orthopedic Surgeons: *Athletic Training and Sports Medicine.* Chicago: AAOS, 1984.
3. American Academy of Orthopedic Surgeons: *Emergency Care and Transportation of the Sick and Injured.* 3rd edition. Chicago: AAOS, 1981.
4. American Medical Association/National Athletic Training Association: *Standard Nomenclature of Athletic Injuries.* Chicago: American Medical Association, 1966.
5. Arnheim DD: *Modern Principles of Athletic Training.* 6th edition. St. Louis: CV Mosby Co., 1985.
6. *Athletic Training.* Winterville, NC. (References to articles herein are written as follows: 6-21:147, which refers to *Athletic Training*—volume 21: page 147.)
7. Booher JM, Thibodeau GA: *Athletic Injury Assessment.* St. Louis: CV Mosby Co., 1985.
8. Daniels L, Worthingham C: *Muscle Testing: Technique of Manual Examination.* Philadelphia: WB Saunders Co., 1972.
9. Downer AH: *Physical Therapy Procedures.* Springfield, IL: Charles C Thomas, 1978.
10. Griffen JE, Karselis TC: *Physical Agents for Physical Therapists.* Springfield, IL: Charles C Thomas, 1978.
11. Harvey J: Rehabilitation of the injured athlete. *Clinics in Sports Medicine* 4: 403-589, 1985.
12. Hoopenfeld S: *Physical Examination of the Spine and Extremities.* New York: Appleton-Century-Crofts, 1976.
13. Kendall HO, Kendall FP, Wadsworth GE: *Muscles: Testing and Function.* Baltimore: Williams & Wilkins, 1971.
14. Knight KL: *Cryotherapy: Theory, Technique, and Physiology.* Chattanooga, TN: Chattanooga Corporation, 1985.
15. Kuland DN: *The Injured Athlete.* Philadelphia: JB Lippincott Company, 1982.
16. Luttgens K, Wells KF: *Kinesiology: Scientific Basis of Human Motion.* Philadelphia: WB Saunders Co., 1985.
17. O'Donoghue DH: *Treatment of Injuries to Athletes.* Philadelphia: WB Saunders Co., 1962.
18. Roy S, Irvin R: *Sports Medicine: Prevention, Evaluation, Management and Rehabilitation.* New Jersey: Prentice-Hall Inc., 1983.

Sources of Information for E and G Modules

The following tables will assist you in studying for Modules E (Taping, Wrapping, Bracing, and Padding) and G (Management of Specific Injuries). The tables are not complete; some entries do not have references, and other sources not listed here may contain material that is equally helpful. However, the tables do provide you an excellent starting point from which to study.

Please help us update and expand this section. If you find errors in the tables or use additional references as you work with the modules, please inform the publisher.

This section is divided into two tables: Table 1 contains references and page numbers for E modules, and Table 2 contains references and page numbers for G modules. The numbers in these tables are cross-references to the texts listed in the recommended resources section.

References described as "Overall" are general information about a specific section of the body; these are then followed by references for specific injuries.

Only the first page number is given in each citation. This system is used to conserve space; always check the following pages to make sure you have read all the pertinent information.

Table 1 E-Module Cross-References for Taping, Wrapping, Bracing, and Padding

Body part	Tape	Wrap	Pad	Brace
Ankle				
Compression		2:91	2:100, 18:391	18:50
Louisiana	2:71, 5:472	18:63		
Illinois	18:61	5:470		
Extra support	2:73			
Open basket	5:476, 18:62			
Closed basket	5:479, 18:335			
Arch				
Longitudinal	5:457, 18:48		5:503, 18:443	
Metatarsal	5:503, 18:60		5:507, 18:409	
Transverse				
Low dye	18:50			
Toes				
Blister				
Hammer	5:509			
Crooked	5:505			
Sprained	18:50			
Heel				
Bruise			5:72	5:455
Spur			5:510	
Lower leg				
Achilles strain	5:482, 18:64			
Shin splints	5:515, 18:65			
Knee				
Compression		2:85, 14:53		
Hyperextension	5:556, 18:66			
Dislocation			5:561	5:561, 18:335
Collateral ligament	5:552, 18:68			5:543, 18:49
Anterior cruciate				18:49
Patellar track			18:48	5:561
Thigh				
Compression		2:82, 5:579	2:81	
Groin				
Adductors	5:595, 18:71			
Rectus femoris				

Body part	Tape	Wrap	Pad	Brace
Low back				
Sacroiliac				
Lumbosacral				5:633
Hip				
Pointer	18:71	5:333	5:337	
Shoulder				
Sling		2:90, 5:327		
Spica		5:331, 18:50		
Sternoclavicular	5:703			
Acromioclavicular	5:705, 18:76		2:97	2:197, 18:177
Glenohumeral	5:709	18:77	2:98	
Elbow				
Contusion		2:48	18:209	
Hyperextension	5:735, 18:75			
Epicondylitis				5:763, 18:224
Forearm				
Splints				
Wrist				
Contusion		5:755		
Flexion	5:753, 18:74	2:98		
Extension	2:61			
Hand				
Contusion	5:755		2:98	
Sprain	2:61, 5:754	5:331	18:49	
Metacarpal fracture	18:87			
Thumb				
Sprain	5:759, 18:72		2:98	
Fingers				
PIP sprain	5:131, 18:237	5:329		
DIP sprain	18:239	5:329		
Boutonniere	18:238			
Dislocation				
Hyperextension	18:72			
Mallet	18:243			5:757

Table 2 G-Module Cross-References for Management of Specific Injuries

Injury	Mechanism	Evaluation	Rehabilitation	Prevention	Taping
G1. Foot					
Overall	7:119	7:188	11:405, 18:133		
Blisters	5:424, 18:407	5:449, 18:407	5:460, 18:407	5:460, 18:407	5:460, 18:407
Calluses and corns	5:424	5:424	18:407	18:407	18:407
Bunion	5:505, 10:209	5:505		5:505	5:505
Ingrown toenail	5:426	18:408	5:426	5:426	
Hammer toe	5:509, 10:220	5:509, 10:220	5:509, 10:220	5:509, 10:220	5:509, 10:220
Neuroma	5:508, 18:405	18:405	18:405	18:405	18:405
Sprained hallux	18:406	18:406	18:406	18:406	5:459, 6-22:215
Sprained digit					
Arch strains	5:457, 14:204	5:457	5:457	5:457	
Fractured metatarsals	5:460				
Plantar fasciitis	5:511, 18:441	18:343	18:343	18:343	6-22:317
Heel bruise	5:455	5:455	5:455	5:455	5:455
Bursitis	18:440	18:440	18:440		
Tenosynovitis					
Fracture phalange	5:459	5:459			
Stress fractures	5:512	5:512			
Avulsion fractures	18:401	18:401	18:401		18:401
Sinus tarsi syndrome	12:216	7:378			
G2. Ankle					
Overall	5:473	7:371	5:483, 11:527	5:467	
1st° ankle sprain	5:473	5:465		5:465	
2nd° ankle sprain	5:477				
3rd° ankle sprain	5:477				
Sprain/dislocation		5:489			
Muscular strain	5:478				
Fractures					
Stress fractures					
Avulsion fractures					
G3. Lower leg					
Overall	5:481, 10:218	7:371, 18:422		18:417	5:481
Achilles tendon strain	5:514, 12:218	6:481, 10:218, 18:379	5:481, 18:379		5:482, 18:64
Achilles tendon bursitis/tenosynovitis	5:515, 18:433	12:218, 18:439			5:15, 18:65
Anterior shin splints	18:433	12:227, 6-24:31	5:515, 18:433		18:403
Posterior shin splints		12:229			

96

(Cont.)

Anterior compartment compression syndrome	5:516, 18:375	6-24:31, 18:436	18:436	18:436	
Muscular strain	5:490	5:490	5:490		6-24:45
Muscular spasm	5:490	5:490	5:490		14:205
Contusions	5:489, 18:375	5:489, 18:375	5:489, 18:375	5:489, 18:375	
Peroneal nerve	18:375	18:375	14:205	14:205	
Fractures	5:492, 18:85	18:85	18:85	14:205	
Stress fractures	5:512				
G4. Knee					
Overall	2:242, 7:396	2:42, 5:530, 7:410	2:298, 5:565, 11:513	5:543	
Torn medial meniscus	2:279, 5:546	2:279, 5:546	5:556		
Torn lateral meniscus	5:546	5:546	5:554		
Cruciate strain anterior	5:545	2:250, 5:545			
Cruciate strain posterior	5:546	5:546			
Medial collateral sprain					
Superficial	5:547	5:547	5:547		5:553
Deep	5:544	5:544	5:544		5:553
Lateral collateral sprain	5:544	5:544	5:544	5:555	5:553
Rotary instability	5:545	2:254			
Bursitis	2:286, 5:547, 7:406		5:547		
Capsular contusion	5:547	5:547			
Contused vastus medialis	5:547				
Patellofemoral joint pain	2:271, 7:408	5:541	5:562		
Patellar tendinitis	2:275, 7:409	5:564			
Patellar tendon rupture	5:564	5:540			
Patellar subluxation	2:275				
Baker's cyst	2:288	5:557	5:558		5:556
Synovial plica					
Hyperextended knee	5:532				
Osgood-Schlatter disease	2:289, 7:409	5:563			
Fractures	2:294, 5:559				
G5. Thigh					
Overall	5:578, 7:444	7:457	5:578		
Quadriceps contusion	7:448	5:578	5:604		
Quadriceps strain	5:582		5:604		
Hamstring strain	5:584, 7:450	5:582			
Femoral fracture	5:580				
Myositis ossificans					
G6. Hip and groin					
Overall	5:589	7:457			
Trochanteric bursitis	5:598				

Table 2 (Continued)

Injury	Mechanism	Evaluation	Rehabilitation	Prevention	Taping
G6. Hip and groin (continued)					
Snapping hip	5:600, 7:455				
Hip sprain	7:456				
Lateral hip pain	18:428				
Hip pointer	5:601, 7:452		5:605		5:602
Dislocated hip	5:599, 7:456, 18:287				
Groin strain	5:594, 18:282	5:594			5:594
Hernia	5:611	5:611			
Pelvic fracture	5:603	5:603			
Iliopsoas bursitis	5:586				
Contused genitalia	18:291				
Spermatic cord torsion	5:615				
Traumatic hydrocele of tunica vaginalis	5:615				
G7. Low back					
Overall	5:613	5:624, 7:289	5:640, 18:281	5:632	
Lumbar sprain/strain	5:633, 18:270	18:270		18:270	
Disk rupture	5:636, 18:275	5:636, 18:275	5:636, 18:275		
Lumbar contusion	5:632	5:632	5:632	5:632	
Lumbosacral sprain/strain	5:634	5:634	5:634	5:634	
Sacroiliac sprain	5:636				
Sciatica	5:633				
Transverse spinous process fracture	5:638				
Spondylolysis	5:637, 18:279	5:637, 18:279	5:637		
Spondylolisthesis	5:637, 18:279	5:637, 18:279	5:637		
Spondylitis	18:279	18:279			
G8. Chest and abdomen					
Overall	2:340, 7:315	7:330			
Rectus abdominis contusion	5:613, 18:290				
Spleen rupture	5:613, 18:291	5:613			
Kidney contusion		5:613			
Liver contusion		5:613			
Stitch in the side	5:612, 7:324				
Wind knocked out	5:612, 18:291				
Rib fracture	5:617, 18:289	5:617	5:617		
Rib contusion	5:617, 18:289				

(Cont.)

Table 2 (Continued)

Injury	Mechanism	Evaluation	Rehabilitation	Prevention	Taping
Forearm (continued)					
Radial head fracture	18:209				
Forearm splints	5:743				
G11. Wrist and hand					
Overall	5:745, 7:547	5:747, 7:556	5:763		
Colles' fracture	5:753	18:233	5:745		
Carpal navicular fracture	5:753, 7:548	5:753, 18:234	5:753	5:745	
Lunate dislocation	7:546	18:235			
Hamate fracture	18:234				
Radioulnar sprain	7:546				
Wrist ganglion	5:752, 7:546	5:752	5:752		
Sprain	5:752	5:752, 7:445	5:752		
Nerve compression					
Hand					
Overall	5:755	7:556	5:763		
Contusion	5:755, 7:554				5:755
Thumb ulnar collateral sprain	5:759, 7:554	18:235	18:235		5:759
PIP sprain	5:759, 18:236	5:759			
Interphalangeal dislocations	5:761, 7:554	18:238			
Boutonniere deformity	5:757, 18:237	5:757, 18:237	5:757		
Mallet finger	5:756, 7:552	5:756, 18:242	5:756		
Metacarpal fractures	5:762, 7:555	18:239			
Phalangeal fractures	5:762	18:241			18:87
Subungual hematoma	5:756, 18:244		18:244		
G12. Head and neck					
Overall	2:393, 5:654, 7:273	5:651, 7:289	5:651, 18:262	5:651, 18:250	
Skull fracture	18:142	18:142			
Concussion	5:664, 18:142	7:243, 18:142			
Intracranial bleeding	5:668, 18:143	18:143			
Cervical fracture	2:406, 7:282		2:406		
Cervical dislocation		5:660	5:660	5:660	
Cervical sprains/strains	7:281	5:657, 6-24:108	5:657	5:657	
Neck contusion	5:657	5:657	5:657		
Burner	7:487, 661	18:258			

G13. Facial injuries

Scalp hematoma	18:142				
Lacerations	5:428, 18:146				
Jaw fracture	5:671, 18:148	7:252			
Jaw dislocation	7:252				
Dental injuries	5:673, 7:260, 18:149	6-24:139	2:412		5:330
Eye foreign body	5:679, 7:263				
Corneal abrasions	5:680, 18:150	7:264			
Lens or iris injury	5:678, 18:151	6-22:207			
Eye chamber hemorrhage	5:678, 18:151	6-22:207			
Detached retina	7:266, 18:152	5:679			
Contact lens lost in eye	7:268		7:268		
Nose bleed	5:675, 18:152	5:675, 7:254	5:675		
Nasal fracture	5:674, 18:152	5:674	5:674	5:184	18:152
Hematoma auris	5:676, 7:257, 18:152				
Ruptured eardrum	5:258, 18:154			18:155	
Swimmer's ear	5:437, 18:155		5:677		
Ear foreign body	5:677		5:677		

G14. Dermatological conditions

Overall	2:486, 5:418	7:119		
Abrasions	7:123	6-23:341		
Blisters	5:424, 7:133		5:424	5:424
Ingrown toenail	5:426		5:426	
Fungal infections	5:423, 7:135	6-24:12	5:426	
Tinea	5:437	5:437	5:437	
Bacterial infections	5:422, 7:134		5:432	
Impetigo	5:432, 7:135		5:422	
Viral infections	5:422, 7:130		5:430	
Herpes	5:430, 7:136	5:430	5:430	
Warts	5:430, 7:136	5:430	5:430	
Sunburn	5:424, 7:137			
Cellulitis	18:500			
Urticaria	18:501			
Dermatitis	2:488, 18:501			
Infestations	2:493, 5:445			

G15. Common illnesses

Colds	5:488, 767		5:488, 767
Streptococcal infections	5:769, 18:489		5:769, 18:489
Infectious mononucleosis	18:491	2:338	
Canker sores	18:489		

(Cont.)

Table 2 (Continued)

Injury	Mechanism	Evaluation	Rehabilitation	Prevention	Taping
G15. Common illnesses (continued)					
Sinusitis	5:768, 18:490				
Bronchitis	18:490				
Hypertension	18:492				
Urine abnormalities	18:493				
Venereal diseases	5:442, 18:494				
Allergies	5:771, 18:495				
Asthma	5:770, 18:496	2:453, 476, 6-24:6			
Diarrhea	5:773				
Constipation	5:772				
Hemorrhoids	5:772				
Appendicitis	5:774				
Indigestion	5:773				
Diabetes	2:473, 5:775		2:473		
Epilepsy	2:460, 5:778		2:460		
Menstrual irregularities	5:779				
Insect stings	2:242				
Shock	2:365		2:365		
Heat illnesses	2:526, 18:477		2:526, 18:477	2:526, 18:477	